Medical Justice

International Healthcare Ethics

Juliet Rothman
General Editor

Vol. 5

PETER LANG
New York • Washington, D.C./Baltimore • Bern
Frankfurt am Main • Berlin • Brussels • Vienna • Oxford

Sara E. Austin

Medical Justice

A Guide to Fair Provision

PETER LANG
New York • Washington, D.C./Baltimore • Bern
Frankfurt am Main • Berlin • Brussels • Vienna • Oxford

Library of Congress Cataloging-in-Publication Data

Austin, Sara E.
Medical justice: a guide to fair provision / Sara E. Austin.
p. cm. — (International healthcare ethics; vol. 5)
Includes bibliographical references.
1. Medical care—Social aspects—United States. 2. Medical economics—Moral and ethical aspects—United States. 3. Right to health care—United States. I. Title. II. Series.
RA445 .A95 362.1′0973—dc21 00-022977
ISBN 0-8204-4935-0
ISSN 1073-5771

Die Deutsche Bibliothek-CIP-Einheitsaufnahme

Austin, Sara E.:
Medical justice: a guide to fair provision / Sara E. Austin.
–New York; Washington, D.C./Baltimore; Bern;
Frankfurt am Main; Berlin; Brussels; Vienna; Oxford: Lang.
(International healthcare ethics; Vol. 5)
ISBN 0-8204-4935-0

The paper in this book meets the guidelines for permanence and durability of the Committee on Production Guidelines for Book Longevity of the Council of Library Resources.

Printed in the United States of America

DEDICATION

For my mother, Virginia Schultz, who taught me the value of completing projects once begun. This book was originally the dissertation required for completion of my Ph.D. In honor of my mother, the oral defense of it took place on her birthday, May 28, 1998.

TABLE OF CONTENTS

PREFACE

It became apparent even before then-Presidential Candidate William Clinton campaigned on health-care reform, that a crisis existed in both the costs and coverage of health care in the United States. With a background in both medical ethics and political philosophy, I became interested in the question of whether any leading political theories were capable of justifying a right to health care in the United States. My research led me to consider several different theoretical approaches to distributive justice, among which were Utilitarianism, Kantianism and Communitarianism. I quickly dispatched of Utilitarianism, for it is notable in its failure to accommodate just distributions in any straightforward way.

Several theorists, including Ronald Green and Norman Daniels, had attempted to extend John Rawls's neo-Kantian theory of justice to health care. Since those fields seemed more fertile, I began digging in them. Those fields yielded some interesting and insightful produce, but they failed to yield a definitive result. I then began digging in the Communitarian field Michael Walzer had planted. His theory, too, offered some interesting fruit, but again, it failed to produce an unblemished result. All three of these commentators had proposed a just solution to the current distribution of health care, yet I found that all three solutions were, themselves, fraught with problems.

In light of these problems, and with their helpful insights in hand, I began approaching the issue of a just distribution of health care from another angle. It occurred to me that health care is distributed in the United States according to a certain pattern. There exists a public distribution of health care (e.g., Medicare and Medicaid), an employment-based distribution of health care, and a private distribution of health care. Upon further reflection, it seemed that each of these distributions were governed by an underlying distributive principle. The question then became, If the obligations implied by these principles were fulfilled in our existing distribution of health care, would the resulting distribution be just?

I thus set out a somewhat idealized version of the existing distribution, and applied that version to cases of health care. It was my belief that if the differences in health care treatments found between the different distributions could be justified by appeal to the underlying principle of each prong, then the distribution would be just if it were applied correctly. I found after consideration of various health care treatments, that the differences in care could be justified by appeal to the various principles underlying each prong of the distribution. I thus conclude that the version of health care delivery I set out is just.

ACKNOWLEDGMENTS

I wish to express my appreciation to Georgia Warnke, without whose insightful suggestions and guidance this book would not exist. Andrews Reath's helpful comments and suggestions, especially in respect to the Rawlsian material, have been invaluable additions.

I wish to thank, as well, the ethics committee at Loma Linda University Medical Center, especially Dr. Robert Orr, for allowing me to join their ethics conferences. Their careful consideration of difficult cases has helped to keep my eye on principled decisions, and my feet planted firmly in the realities of medical care. I also wish to express my appreciation to Norman Daniels for his prompt and helpful responses to questions that arose while I was researching his theory. Robert Clinton has donated technological support; I am grateful for his computer expertise. Kerrin McMahan has provided invaluable editorial expertise. If there remain any typographical or grammatical errors in the text, I must claim responsibility.

A special word of appreciation goes to Allison Shalinsky without whose generous advice, encouragement, and continuous presence this project would not have been completed. I have incurred a debt to her that is impossible to repay; she has my most sincere gratitude. There are some people whom we tend never to forget. I believe they are, for the most part, the ones who pass on to us valuable lessons that, in our better moments, we hope to pass on to others.

CHAPTER 1

INTRODUCTION

The distribution of health care has been, and continues to be, a problem for those concerned with distributive justice. At the heart of the present debate in the United States is the question of whether considerations of justice require the government to insure that its citizens have access to health care. This question leads to further questions: if the government is obligated, for what kinds of health care is it responsible? Further, how much health care should a government thus obligated provide? It is here that difficult choices must be made. We must make choices among different kinds and amounts of health care when not all who may benefit will be treated.

There are several directions from which one might enter the debate. One might argue that the distribution of health care lies outside the realm of governmental or social concern, and so it is not a concern of social justice. Alternatively, one might argue for a variety of reasons—including the claims that since health care treatments significantly affect the prospects and well-being of individuals living in a community, or that citizens need health care in order to realize the other benefits of society—that it is a concern of social justice. There exists a third possibility for approaching the debate: namely, that some health-care treatments are a social concern, while others are merely a matter of individual preference.

Several bases upon which one might adopt the first candidate suggest themselves. One might have in mind the idea that the government should play a minimal role in the lives of its citizens. Or one might have certain ideas about the relation between justice and the state of one's health. For instance, one's religious beliefs might be such that the state of one's health properly lies in the hands of God and not the government. For those not arguing on religious grounds, the claim might be that since no injustice has been perpetrated, the notion of justice is irrelevant. Hence, individuals may have some unspecified duty to aid those in need, but there exists no governmental obligation based in justice to insure access to health care.

If one thinks that health care is a concern of social justice, then again several bases for this idea suggest themselves. For instance, one might think that government ought to play an expanded role in the lives of its citizens, i.e., that it has certain responsibilities for providing at least some of the means by which citizens have an equal chance to participate in the benefits of the society to which they belong. These benefits might include an equal chance to hold certain positions, or engage in educational pursuits or desirable life styles, or more broadly, the ability to equally participate in the civil and political freedoms offered by our society, all of which might be impossible without first having equal access to health care.

Both of these alternatives involve theories of distributive justice. The first involves a libertarian, or at least a minimal state, theory, while the second involves a liberal egalitarian theory. Each moves from different theoretical perspectives to claims about what justice either does or does not require. But they seem to justify both too much and too little. For instance, if one starts from a minimal state perspective, the claim might be that one of the few legitimate responsibilities of government is the provision of protection, but not health care. Yet, if lack of health care adversely affected that provision, this claim may justify less then the libertarian wants. Might not the libertarian say in this special case that government has a responsibility to provide health care? On the other hand, if one starts from the liberal egalitarian point of view, the claim may be that since equality is a fundamental political and moral precept in the US, then everyone ought to have equal access to whatever health-care treatments are available. Yet, the liberal egalitarian may find this claim justifies too much. It is not necessarily the case that all health care treatments give rise to claims based in justice. Some cosmetic treatments seem to be clear instances of personal preference rather than instances of justice. Hence, the liberal egalitarian may want to impose constraints on a claim based upon a principle of equality if it is to be a reasonable one.

We might, then, want to consider a third possibility: that some health care is a matter of social justice, i.e., claims to health care might be made on the basis of a broad sense of equal opportunity to participate both in the good of health care and the other benefits offered by the US which health care affords. Some health care, on the other hand, is more a matter of personal preferences; i.e., some treatments are quite outside the domain of a social obligation. And still other treatments occupy a middle ground between the first two. Since I think it is this possibility that is embodied by our actual practices, I want to examine the existing distribution of health care in the United States and consider whether it, or some modification of it, can be justified. I shall proceed in this chapter by assembling a description of our existing distribution of health care and discussing various problems it raises.

I do not want to dismiss out of hand, however, the insights offered by theories of justice spun for the distinct good of health care. These theories provide deep insights into what sort of good health care is, how health care is related to questions of justice, and the many problems associated with formulating a just distribution. To that end, Chapters Two and Three will consider Ronald Green's[1] and Norman Daniels's[2] extensions of John Rawls's theory of distributive justice.[3] In contrast to the liberal egalitarian bases of these two extensions, Chapter Four will examine the communitarian theory offered by Michael Walzer.[4] These theorists advance systematic criticisms of the existing distribution and offer alternatives to it for our consideration. However, I believe that these alternatives, themselves, are fraught with problems. In their respective chapters, I shall address these problems. In Chapter Five I want to give a somewhat idealized model under which a version of our existing distribution is defensible. And in Chapter Six, I conclude by applying the model to troubling cases of health care and show how they might be resolved in a just way.[5]

The Existing Distribution of Health Care

Total US health care expenditures in the US for 1994 were approximately $900 billion.[6] There are several ways one might slice that $900 billion. One might ascertain how much was spent on environmentally caused diseases, or on heart related diseases. Or, one might obtain the data on how much was spent by one segment of the population. Or, one might divide the $900 billion by locality. But I rather want to concentrate on the way provision of health care is funded. There are, I believe, three roughly distinct parts. One division I shall call the private provision of health care, one division I shall call the employment-based provision, and one I shall call public provision. The first division constitutes approximately 21 per cent (or $189 billion) of the total expenditures, the second division approximately 30 per cent (or $271 billion), and the last division approximately 48 percent (or $433 billion). The members making up each division shift from time to time, but the divisions themselves remain fairly stable.

By the private provision of health care I mean that division in which the members either pay for their health care out of pocket, or pay for their entire health-care insurance. This division, itself, is divided into two groups. The more fortunate members of this group might be thought of as free agents with respect to contracting for health care. Their ability to access health care is dependent solely on how much they are willing to spend out-of-pocket for medical care and insurance, and how much health care providers are willing to sell. Insurance companies typically turn a profit by limiting the kinds and amounts of health service to which their subscribers have access. But the more fortunate members of this group are not necessarily subject to any one set of insurance rules governing collective access to health care since they can buy whatever exotic care or insurance they want or need. Hence, we can expect them to receive more kinds and amounts of health care than others whether it is medically appropriate or not. To this extent, members of this part of the privately insured division have access to just about any health care they desire because they have the ability to pay for it.

Access for less fortunate members of this group is limited by their ability to make out-of-pocket payments, or purchase insurance. These members typically will shop around for insurance plans that best suit their needs, given their resources. Since they can rarely afford more than one plan, we can expect them to be subject to one set of insurance rules, thus limiting the kinds and amounts of health care to which they have access. For instance, they may have hospital costs and physician fees covered, but not the costs of prescription drugs or dental care. Hence, these members are entitled to some set of health care—hopefully what they most need—but not necessarily everything they need. Thus, within this one division, access is differentially distributed according to ability to pay.

By employment-based provision, I mean that access to health care in which members have their health care insurance paid for either fully or partially by their employer. Here, too, there exists a variety of plans. Some employers may provide their employees with a fairly hefty package of health care benefits. For instance, the package may include catastrophic illness, hospitalization, doctor's fees, nursing care, prescription drugs, eye care and dental care. Within this group, some employees have the whole package paid for by their employer, and some may have to contribute from their paychecks a portion of their insurance premiums.

Other employers provide an insurance plan that covers much less health care. It may cover only doctors' fees, hospitalization, and some percent of prescriptions. Then again, it may cover doctors' fees, eye care, and hospitalization for only some conditions, or for some specialists. Here again, it may be the case that employers pay for only some of the premium, while employees contribute, as well. Within this group, some employees may find it necessary to purchase health care insurance other than what is provided by the employer in order to meet their specific needs. Sometimes there still exists the choice of a traditional indemnity plan in which one's doctor is paid on a fee-for-service basis by the insurance company. Much more prevalent now are different managed care plans (HMOs) because they focus on containing costs while increasing services. Hence, the kinds of health care provided by employment-based schemes vary from employer to employer, as well as within any one firm. Thus, within this rough division there are a variety of health care plans and a variety of payment plans, from which follows differential access to health care, just as in the first division. So, members of this group are entitled to that health care which is offered by the plans chosen by their employers, and what they can afford over and above that provided by their employers.[7]

By public provision of health care, I mean that group whose members receive health care through Medicare, Medicaid, and state and county funding. President Truman first sponsored the Medicare Program in 1945. In 1965 it, along with Medicaid, was legislated into law under President Johnson as part of his Great Society programs. Prior to the passage of Medicaid and Medicare, a patchwork of programs sponsored by state and local governments, charities, and community hospitals financed and provided scattered, mostly emergency health care services to some indigent Americans.[8] Medicare was enacted as a social-insurance program in contrast to a welfare program;[9] it was designed as a security net to insure health care to people upon retirement. In 1966, 19.1 million elderly people were covered by Medicare insurance; that figure grew to about 33 million people (or 12.8 percent of the population) in 1994.[10] In addition, more than 4 million disabled Americans and 200,000 Americans with end-stage renal disease are covered by Medicare even though they are under sixty-five, enabling them to receive essential health services that many could not otherwise afford.[11]

Under Part A of the Medicare plan, beneficiaries receive hospital insurance, which is financed through payroll taxes on current employers and workers. Under Part B, people can elect supplemental coverage for physician and outpatient services. General tax revenues provide about 65 percent of the funding for Part B while 31 percent comes from the premiums paid by beneficiaries and the rest from interest income.

While there is no single basic benefit package, the Medicare program covers most inpatient hospital costs for which beneficiaries must meet small deductibles and copayments. Part B covers outpatient hospital services, physician fees, home health care, short stays in skilled nursing facilities, hospices, renal dialysis and medical equipment such as wheelchairs. It also includes some preventive services such as mammograms, Pap smears and certain vaccines. However, it normally does not include many preventive treatments such as annual physicals, eye or ear exams, other immunizations, and long-term nursing home care. Nor does it include prescription drugs or dental care. Even with Medicare Parts A and B and Medigap coverage,[12] the elderly spend an average of 14 percent of their after-tax incomes on health care. Hence, for the Medicare group, both public policy and ability to pay determine access to health care.

The Medicaid Program, on the other hand, was enacted as a joint federal/state welfare program to provide health care insurance to low-income Americans. In the early 1970s, the proportion of the population covered by Medicaid was 8 percent. That figure has risen to 13 percent, or 34 million Americans. In 1994, Medicaid expenditures were $135.5 billion, constituting 6 percent of federal outlays (or only 10 percent of federal entitlement spending, compared to, e.g., 40 percent for Social Security and 20 percent for Medicare), and only 13.3 percent of state general fund outlays (compared to 33.8 percent toward elementary and secondary education).[13]

For those Americans eligible to receive Medicaid, benefits include physician fees, hospital costs, and nursing facility services, eye care, dental care, and prescription drugs. Most states also include physical therapy, hospice care, and a variety of rehabilitative services. About half of the states provide screening, prevention, and diagnostic services for adults, and chiropractic and occupation therapy.[14]

Before President Clinton signed The Personal Responsibility and Work Opportunity Act of 1996,[15] there was a federal guarantee that US residents with low incomes and meager financial resources had access to a decent package of health care. Among this group are impoverished children under the age of six (nearly 17 million, or one in four American children) and pregnant women if their incomes are below 133 per cent of the federal poverty threshold ($10,030). Long-term nursing home care, prescription drugs, and other services not covered by Medicare are provided for the low-income elderly (about 3.8 million) as well as deductibles and premiums for Medicare benefits. The 1988 Family Support Act extended Medicaid coverage to more low-income Americans who have jobs without health coverage. Medicaid also provides coverage for approximately 5.4 million Americans who are disabled or blind. These individuals qualify for benefits due to low incomes and minimal assets, or because they have medical expenses that consume most of their incomes. In addition, Medicaid provides benefits for nearly 40 percent of patients with AIDS at some point during their illness. And finally, thirty-six states have elected to provide Medicaid to people who qualify as "medically needy." These people do not qualify based on their income and assets, but they are accepted because they face huge medical bills. The average income for eligibility for this population is 53 percent of the poverty level. Thus the health care to which the Medicaid members of this group are entitled is dependent on qualifying for benefits.

What seems obvious from this discussion, then, is that the provision of health care in the US varies both among and within groups. But is there anything wrong with that? My question is, Can the three-pronged provision of health care in the US, or some version of it, be defended? It seems to me that a defense must rely on some sort of an appeal to differences among groups, rather than differences within groups. And, indeed, Aristotle first articulated a general principle of equality stating that equals ought to be treated equally and unequals ought to be treated unequally to explain when differences in treatment are justified. So we might think that his formal (or general) principle of equality justifies the variability in access to health care. By itself, however, it does not get us very far in explaining the differences, for it fails to specify the relevant respects in which differences between individuals justifies differences in access. Typically, when we are attempting to explain differences in treatment, we draw on relevant differences between groups or individuals to justify differential treatment. Now, one reason to think that the existing distribution might be defensible is that the individuals whose health care is provided under these different prongs generally do not occupy equal positions in our society. For the most part, those whose health care is publicly provided are in the lower economic bracket, and those whose health care is employment based typically are in a middle income position, although they may be in either a high or a low income bracket, as well. And those who provide for their own health care are normally in an upper income bracket. We might think, then, that these differences in positions justify differences in health care treatment. This explanation for the differences in treatment, however, has obvious exceptions. For instance, many people who receive Medicare are in the upper income bracket. And many who are either employed or unemployed are in the low-income bracket, yet they receive neither publicly funded nor employment-based health care. The first exception might not worry us too much provided it did not have an effect on the low-income group.[16] But the latter exception might worry us quite a bit, for the members of this group are ineligible for any coverage unless they can fund it themselves. Moreover, these exceptions fail to articulate differences that are relevant to differential treatment; i.e., most of the members of these latter two groups need health care, but it is not provided, nor is it likely they can afford to pay for the kinds they need. Thus, one reason to think the three-pronged provision of health care might be indefensible is the gaps within each division.

Gaps in Health Care Provision

About 42 percent of Americans living in poverty are not covered by

Medicaid. In 1994, the total population with no health insurance was 17.3 percent, or about 40 million people.[17] Most of those uninsured poor do not qualify because they have no children, they are not disabled, and they are not pregnant. For instance, in a two-parent family with one parent working full time, only the children are eligible for coverage unless the mother is pregnant. Thus, the Medicaid program which is supposed to insure health care for the poor covered only slightly more than half the poor in 1994.

Before the passage of the new welfare Act, persons eligible for AFDC were automatically entitled to Medicaid coverage. The Act severs this automatic link and amends it to say that any reference to eligibility under AFDC shall mean the state's AFDC state plan as it existed on July 16, 1996. A state can modify those "frozen" plans in three ways: it can lower its income standards; it can increase income or resource standards and medically needy income levels; and it may use income and resource methodologies that are less restrictive than the methodologies used under the state plan as of July 16, 1996. In addition, states will have the option of denying Medicaid coverage to persons who are legal residents but not citizens and new immigrants will be automatically barred for five years after entry. If states exercise their options to reduce coverage, and new immigrants are automatically barred for five years, it seems reasonable to conclude that less than half the poor will be insured under Medicaid.

Several states, for instance California and New York, require by law that counties pick up the health care tab for indigents who otherwise are not funded. But counties, themselves, are having difficulty meeting their responsibilities due to huge budget deficits. In 1996, Los Angeles county laid off 4,187 health care workers, and plans to close 28 of its 39 community health centers and five of its six comprehensive health centers which together serve more than 1 million poor, working uninsured and the elderly.[18] This situation will not be improved by the Act Clinton signed in 1996. In addition to the above mentioned provisions of the Act, the federal government bars illegal immigrants from receiving most federal and state welfare benefits and gives much more leeway to states to designate who is eligible for Medicaid. For instance, it gives states the right to choose whether legal immigrants are eligible for Medicaid and allows states to deny Medicaid coverage to an adult who loses welfare benefits by not going to work. Hence, the county agencies, which have been called last-resort programs for indigent people, and which are already financially over-burdened, will not receive federal funds to pick up the tab, and depending on legislative action, they may not have the state funds to do it either. It is thus likely that the counties will be unable to fill the gaps left by Medicaid.

In addition, 10 to 20 percent of the population, or 25 million to 48 million, less than 65 years of age with either privately funded or employment-based insurance are underinsured.[19] This group consists mostly of individuals working in low-paying jobs which provide few health care benefits. The 1988 Family Support Act extended Medicaid benefits to the children of families in this group. However, as already noted, able-bodied adults qualify for these benefits in only about 36 states where provisions have been made for the "medically needy." According to several articles,[20] it is these patients who have trouble paying their health care bills. With less funding from the federal government, and a greater burden placed on state and county programs, it's unclear how these individuals will get their health needs met. It is difficult to give exact numbers for the uninsured and underinsured. But figuring conservatively, 27.3 to 37.3 percent of the population, or 65 to 88 million people living in the US either have no health care insurance or are underinsured.

We started this discussion by noting that there are three sources by which health care is funded: private provision, employment-based provision and public provision. The implication is that among these three sources most people will have access to the social good of health care. But the data show that approximately one third of all people living in America either do not have access, or have limited access. Moreover, these figures were compiled before the provisions of the Personal Responsibility and Work Opportunity Act of 1996 came into effect. We have no way of knowing how state legislatures will determine Medicaid eligibility based on the Act, but it seems likely that upwards of 8 million more people will lose benefits under reform proposals.[21] Thus, any assumption that the three-pronged provision of health care covers most Americans is false.

Principles Involved in the Existing Distribution of Health Care

A second reason to think that the existing distribution is indefensible is that health care is a single good, but it is governed by different distributive principles. For instance, the first way in which differences in access to health care has been shown is that some people have the ability to pay for some or all of their health care needs. This ability is expressed by a free market principle which embodies the claim that in a free society people ought to have the right to accumulate and dispose of their property in any way they wish so long as no laws are violated and no one is harmed. So if buyers have the ability and desire to purchase health care, and providers are willing to sell it, then these exchanges should not be interfered with.

A second way in which differences in access has been noted is that many people have their health insurance provided by their employer. Here it seems the connection between health care provision and a specified principle of justice is more vague. Perhaps it is vague because it is unclear what the link between insurance and employment is. Employers first provided health insurance during World War II when the government froze wages and prices. To attract and keep employees, firms had to offer something that evaded the wage controls. So they offered pensions and health insurance. In addition, government has encouraged this policy by providing tax breaks to employers when they pay for their employee's health insurance.[22] Yet as Eric Banfield has pointed out, employers do not provide fire or auto insurance. So in order to discover the link between health insurance and employment, it seems we first have to say what might be special about health care that does not pertain to fire or auto insurance. Clearly health care keeps employees more healthy and able to contribute to the production of goods and services in America. It may very well be that employment-based provision of health care is grounded upon the idea that differences in treatment are justified in order to promote the health of workers, which in turn allows them to contribute to the economic well being of both the company for which they work, and to society in general. In other words, health care ultimately acts as a reward for their contribution to society. Thus, a more specific principle of justice regulating employment-based provision of health care may be the idea that the nation needs healthy workers who contribute to the well being of society, and in consideration of their contribution, they deserve to be rewarded.

The third way in which health care is provided is by public policy. It is tempting to say that the principle underlying this provision is a principle of need. In fact, several philosophers make such a claim. Michael Walzer claims that the communal understanding of health care has already made it a good that should be provided on the basis of need, and that it should be provided equally to all members of the community.[23] And Bernard Williams claims that "the proper ground of distribution of medical care is ill health: this is a necessary truth ... It is a matter of logic that particular sorts of needs [such as ill health] constitute a reason for receiving particular sorts of goods [health care]."[24] However, the principle of need does not sufficiently distinguish health care provision in the public realm from provision in either the private or the employment-based realms. In all three divisions, need plays a significant role. Employees *need* health care provision as much as the unemployed or the wealthy, yet their access to it is differentially provided. So I do not believe that the notion of need, *simpliciter*, provides the appropriate, or definitive distinction among the different provisions.

I want to suggest that what distinguishes public provision of health care from the other provisions is the idea of equal opportunity for all residents of the US to enjoy the good of health care and the benefits derived from it. Some of those benefits include decreased suffering, prevention of ill health and restoration to functioning capacity, as well as providing the opportunity to pursue individual goals. All provisions provide these functions, but I believe that what most distinguishes public provision from the others is the opportunity to compete for jobs, careers and desirable positions offered by our society. The principle of equal opportunity seems to cover a rather broad range of reasons for providing public health insurance, but it will do, I believe, as a reasonably sufficient rubric.

Each of these principles is a specification of Aristotle's principle of formal equality. They are meant to explain the important, relevant respects in which differences in treatment are justified. People who can privately afford to pay for their own health care have more freedom to choose the kinds and amounts of health care they want, as well as more choice in doctors. That is, need, prevention and personal preferences are options for wealthy individuals. Employees get most of their ill-health needs met, as well as some prevention and some personal preferences. But there are limitations on the kinds and amounts of health care, as well as a choice of doctors, depending on the plan chosen by their employer and the plans that they can afford to supplement their benefit package. In the public domain, further limitations are imposed. Ill health is almost always covered, but preventive treatments are not as available, especially for Medicare and Medicaid beneficiaries. Nor do either Medicare, Medicaid or state and local agencies provide treatments which can be thought of as "personal preference" treatments. In addition, fewer doctors accept Medicaid patients,[25] so the choice of doctors is limited.

The upshot of this discussion seems to be this: there seem to be three principles underlying our existing distribution—the ability to pay; merit or desert because of contributing to social well being; and equal opportunity—and these principles seem to correspond to the three divisions of health care provision.

The opponent to various principles governing the distribution of health care might claim that since the subject under discussion is a single good, it should be governed by a single principle. For instance, the opponent of the three-pronged approach to provision of health care may be claiming that health care is no different from other commodities, and so the distribution of all of it should be based on the ability to pay. Other opponents may make similar claims about the principles of need, contribution and equal opportunity. And still others may claim that it is a quite different principle or theory that ought to govern the distribution of health care. Many of these claims seem *prima facie* defensible. Yet, I think we can rule out the principle of need for two reasons. First, it fails to make the finer-grained distinctions among the different prongs of the existing distribution. And second, not all health-care treatments are needs in a strict sense. Rather, some treatments such as cosmetic surgery seem to be clear instances of personal preferences.

Furthermore, I believe that we can rule out a free market principle as the sole principle of distribution. I have already argued that not even a thoroughgoing libertarian would claim that treating health care solely as a commodity would justify as much health care as he might want. If the protection of the state depended on a healthy militia and police force, then surely a theorist of this persuasion would make an exception to treating health care only on the basis of the ability to pay.

Much more interesting, I believe, are the various attempts to unify the distribution of health care under what might broadly be called an equal opportunity principle. In the next chapter, I shall consider Ronald Green's defense of health care based on the idea of it being a social good equal in importance to basic freedoms and liberties. His claim in this regard is that providing health care equally to everyone is as important to realizing individual plans of life as freedoms such as speech, voting and other political liberties. I shall continue in the third chapter with Norman Daniels's theory of health care in which he defends a specific principle of equal opportunity as the correct principle of health care distribution. He does not claim, as Green does, that equal access to health care is as important as political liberties. Rather, Daniels finds an important relationship between equal opportunity and the ability to pursue life plans. In the fourth chapter, I shall investigate a proposed solution to the health care debate advanced by Michael Walzer. His solution, too, might be broadly characterized as an attempt to realize equal opportunity. But rather than an equal opportunity to pursue individual life plans, he is more concerned with an opportunity for citizens to realize equal membership status in their community. I shall argue in these chapters, however, that each attempt to resolve the health care debate is itself fraught with problems. In view of these problems, I shall suggest in the fifth chapter that we return to the existing three-pronged distribution of health care and sketch a somewhat idealized version of it, under which the distribution of health care might be defensible. In the final chapter, I shall apply this idealized version to troublesome cases of health care to see if it coheres both with our moral intuitions about health care and with the principles which I have argued underlie our present distribution.

CHAPTER 2

LIBERAL EGALITARIAN APPROACHES TO HEALTH CARE: GREEN'S PROPOSAL

One of the most deeply held values on a liberal egalitarian approach to distributive justice is the idea of self-determination. That is, it is the belief of liberal egalitarians that human lives go best when they are lived 'from the inside.' Rather than the state (or some other entity) determining our ends or life plans, we demonstrate our respect for the rational capacities of humans when they are given the freedoms and liberties to choose plans of life for which they are most suited and in which they are most interested. There is divergence, however, among egalitarians from this starting point. Some believe that the least amount of interference from government is the best way to achieve the value of self-determination. Others believe that more government assistance is required in order to allow individuals the pursuit of their ends. For instance, the libertarian resists the idea of redistributing money to fund programs for those who are less well off, preferring instead to let most social goods be governed by the ability to pay. On the other hand, egalitarians of the Rawlsian persuasion tend to underwrite the value of self-determination by accommodating the intuition that government ought to play a role in providing more of the means by which people can realize their own ends.[1]

Ronald Green is among this second group.[2] He selects certain core features of a Rawlsian theory of justice, and then extends them in his argument for a right to universal access to health care in the US. His claim in this regard concerns the idea that equal access to health care is as important to insuring the pursuit of life plans as basic political and civil liberties. In this chapter, I shall first set out Green's explication of the elements of Rawls' theory that he considers crucial to his proposal for health care. I shall then show how Green extends Rawlsian justice to include a right to equal access to health care. Following that, I shall discuss various problems that arise from Green's proposal, itself a criticism of the existing distribution of health care.

Green begins his discussion by noting that Rawls sets up a hypothetical social contract situation as a device to make 'vivid' certain values basic to a liberal democracy such as ours. The hypothetical contract situation is basically a thought experiment in which hypothetical persons choose the principles that will govern the basic structure of their society. Rawls calls this hypothetical situation the 'original position' of equality. According to Rawls, liberal democracies are grounded on the twin ideas of individual freedom and equality. By equality, Rawls means parties to the original position have an equal voice, or have the same rights, in choosing the process by which the principles will be chosen: "each can make proposals, submit reasons for their acceptance, and so on."[3] By freedom, Rawls means that each person would be guaranteed certain basic liberties that underwrite their ability to choose reasonable life plans within the political framework they establish in the original position. He thus asks what sort of principles would free and equal individuals choose to govern their social cooperation in a democracy. In order to insure the ideas of equality and freedom, Rawls imposes several constraints and conditions on the original position as parties contract for the principles that will govern their relations.

First, parties to the original position are thought to be rational in the minimal sense, i.e., they are capable of choosing the best means to achieve their ends. Second, they are placed behind a veil of ignorance. They know neither to which society they belong, nor their position in that society; nor do they possess knowledge of their particular desires and preferences. Nor do they possess knowledge of their natural attributes. They possess knowledge neither of their intelligence level nor of their physical advantages or disadvantages. Hence, the veil of ignorance prevents parties from choosing principles of social cooperation that will advantage them in the distribution of social goods. For instance, since parties do not know whether they might turn out to be 90-pound weaklings, it would be irrational for them to choose a distribution in which the most desirable social goods redound to Arnold Schwarzenegger-type individuals. Choosing the terms of social cooperation from behind a veil of ignorance accomplishes two tasks: it produces principles that are impartial to any particular life plan and it greatly simplifies moral reasoning. We only need to ask how any reasonable individual similarly situated would set up a political framework in which she had the best prospects for success.

According to Rawls, the principles chosen in this initial situation will best secure the primary social goods Rawls supposes people will want more of rather than less. These social goods are constituted by political and civil liberties and rights, opportunities, income and wealth and the social bases of self-respect, each of which are thought of as "all-purpose" means to individual life plans. That is, they are goods that normally have a use whatever a person's rational plan of life. Hence, the principles chosen by the parties are

> 1. Each person is to have an equal right to the most extensive total system of equal basic liberties compatible with a similar system of liberty for all, and
> 2. Social and economic inequalities are to be arranged so that they are both: (a) to the greatest benefit of the least advantaged, and (b) attached to offices and positions open to all under conditions of fair equality of opportunity.

Part (a) of the second principle is known as the difference principle, and part (b) is known as the fair equality of opportunity principle.

In addition, Rawls assigns lexical priority to the principles in order to give systematic guidance in their application to the basic institutions of society. The first principle has priority over the second principle and part (b) of the second principle has priority over part (a). Thus, the first principle must be satisfied before the equal opportunity principle, and the equal opportunity principle must be satisfied before the difference principle. Liberties cannot be traded for greater opportunities, nor can opportunities be sacrificed for the sake of greater benefits to the least advantaged. While there are roughly equivalent rights to the basic liberties and opportunity, the difference principle allows inequalities in income and wealth, so long as the least well off do better under this system than under another they might have chosen from the original position.

In his argument from the original position for these principles, Rawls insists that parties will employ maximin reasoning. Maximin reasoning simply means that parties will choose principles which maximize their access to primary social goods should they be among the worst off in society. For example, if one were among a racial minority and discrimination were advantaging to the majority, then the possibility of losing important freedoms and opportunities might be great. Since these losses would be devastating to any life plan, parties would choose principles that maximize minimum expectations. This is a best-worst method of deciding; it asserts that when the chances of winning or losing a greater share of primary goods are unknown, rational agents will use a choice procedure that is rationally prudent and which will result in roughly equal rights to access the primary social goods. Hence, for Rawls the implications of freedom and equality are the following. Freedom is the ability to choose reasonable life plans freely, guaranteed by the basic liberties that the parties have established. Equality does not mean that individuals possess an equal share of material goods. Rather, it means that individuals equally possess the basic liberties and opportunity required to pursue life plans they find most desirable, and for which they are best suited. Thus, Rawls claims that parties to the original position will choose principles that give equal consideration to freely chosen, rational plans of life.

There are several noteworthy aspects of this description for our purposes. First, Rawls does not incorporate any of the specified principles of distributive justice directly into his theory of justice. It is not the case that he rules them out altogether, but rather that his theory is meant to apply to the basic structure of society. As such, it is his contention that principles of need, merit, contribution to society, ability to pay and so on, are inappropriate as first principles of justice. Rawls argues that it is in light of the rights and duties determined by the basic structure of society that citizens have legitimate expectations of well-being. That is, the principles which individuals, regarded as free and equal moral persons, would adopt as the fair terms of social cooperation are the ones that determine legitimate claims to the goods produced and distributed by that society. Hence, justice as fairness "does not interpret the primary problem of distributive justice as one of allocative justice."[4] That is, because of the role of procedural justice, it is not a question of deciding how to allocate a fixed stock of goods. Rather, the issue is setting up a fair social process that determines legitimate expectations. Another way of putting the point is this: if Rawls is correct that the fundamental values in a democratic society are freedom and equality, and that the principles he argues follow from these values are correct, then there are prior claims on the primary goods created and distributed by the terms of social cooperation in virtue of the choices parties have already made by a just procedure in the original position.

However, claims Rawls, specified—or as he calls them, allocative—principles deal with already existing goods for which no one has a prior claim in *justice*. This, of course, does not mean there are no other bases upon which to distribute the existing goods in a society, nor does it mean that the list of primary social goods exhausts the goods about which people have an interest. There are more determinate goods that result from social life, claims to which are determined by specific interactions and transactions in which people engage. To take two examples, the distribution of blood on the battlefield seems appropriately determined on the basis of need and the distribution of luxury cars on the basis of the free market. But these goods, Rawls claims, are not directly distributed by the social structure to which citizens have given prior agreement. They are, rather, only indirectly distributed by the basic structure. Nor do individuals benefiting from these allocations "stand in any existing cooperative relations." If we look only at these particular allocations to identifiable persons "with known desires and needs," we are not yet in a position to judge the justice of the basic structure with which a theory of justice ought to be concerned, according to Rawls. Particular individuals may very well enter into fair trades with each other as contingent circumstances arise, but that fact tells us nothing about the overall structure of society, nor would it determine what free and equal people would accept as the fair terms of social cooperation. Hence, allocative principles are at the wrong level of generality to be considered as first principles of justice.

Moreover, Rawls insists that adopting allocative principles as first principles would inevitably result in conflict between the principles and give us contrary directives. It is appropriate to distribute, e.g., blood on the battlefield on the basis of need, and similarly with the distribution of luxury cars on the basis of ability to pay. But a theory of distributive justice is much broader in scope. Do we distribute rights and liberties on the basis of need? or on ability to pay? or on some other basis? Without some way of systematically organizing the distribution of goods made available by social cooperation, we will end up with a jumble of competing claims and principles with no practical guidelines because there are no priority rules that unify them under a general theory.

Second, it should be noted that Rawls distinguishes the social primary goods from the natural primary goods. Natural goods include attributes such as intelligence, physical strength and health, imagination and natural skills and talents. Rawls focuses primarily on the social goods because, he argues, they are directly distributed by social institutions, while natural goods are only indirectly distributed by them, if they are distributed by them at all. For the most part, Rawls claims that natural goods are "distributed" by nature, rather than by society.

However, both Rawls's fair equality of opportunity principle and the difference principle are designed to respond to our moral intuitions that individuals should not suffer the consequences of social and natural inequalities for which they are not responsible. That is, both principles are supposed to make a distinction between the choices we make and our circumstances. The fair equality of opportunity principle mitigates social inequalities by insuring a fair competition for income, power, authority and prestige to those from the lower social classes and minorities. At the same time, Rawls tries to accommodate inequalities in natural goods by the difference principle. By this principle, the more unfortunate will not be disadvantaged in the distribution of social goods because of circumstances over which they have no control. For instance, some individuals will be less talented, less resourceful, less skillful and less healthy than their fellow citizens. The difference principle is designed to mitigate natural inequalities for which we are not responsible, not by attempting to do away with them, but by insuring a decent income level to the less naturally advantaged. They will, of course, still be less fortunate due to their natural limitations, but according to Rawls, since their expectations have been maximized, these inequalities are now justifiable to them.

Finally, it should be emphasized that Rawls gives priority to equal liberties and opportunity over differences in income and wealth, i.e., he allows inequality in the distribution of material goods but not in liberties and opportunity. He is, in effect, arguing that the important social good of self-respect relies more on rights, liberties and opportunity and less on the equal distribution of income and wealth. "The basis of self-esteem in a just society is not then one's income share but the publicly affirmed distribution of fundamental rights and liberties."[5] In part, this view is motivated by the idea that greater liberties and opportunity allow for the free exchange of ideas and the development of ways of life that are essential to pursuing life plans judged valuable to the person who lives that life. More importantly, when society creates equal basic liberties and equal opportunity, it affirms everyone's equal worth. That is the social basis of self-respect.

Green's Extension of Rawlsian Justice

With these elements of Rawls's theory in place, Green marshals his defense of a right to health care based on Rawls's contract theory. He argues that parties to the original position would use maximin reasoning to arrive at a separate principle of equal access to health care because it is "a value all rational agents would want, whatever their other values."[6] However, it is not always clear whether Green means access to health care is the value all rational agents would want, or whether he means health, itself, is the value. He sometimes speaks of health, itself, as a primary social good: "This is not the general question of the relative place of health among the primary goods, but the more complicated one of how far a general priority should be carried out."[7] At other times he speaks of health as a socially desirable objective to be secured by the primary social good of access to health care: "[T]here is the question of how extensive the health care services of a society should be, and what priorities a society should establish between health and other socially desirable objectives."[8] And at yet other times, he implies that health has its importance because it secures the primary social good of self-respect: "Even more apparently than governmental interference, disease and ill health interfere with our happiness and undermine our self-confidence and self-respect."[9]

In Rawlsian terms, if Green means health as a primary social good, then presumably he means it as one of the "all-purpose means" which secures desirable goals of rational agents, much like basic liberties and opportunities secure goals. And if he means health in the second sense as a socially desirable objective, then it seems to be a goal, in itself, which society is to promote by creating a right to access health care. But if he means it in the third sense, then health gains its importance because it protects the important social good of self respect which, in turn, gives people the confidence to pursue their own goals. Thus, there are three ways we can understand the significance Green gives to health: as an all-purpose means to individual goals, as a goal of society, or as just one among many goods which helps promote the important social good of self-respect.

There is yet a fourth way to understand Green's discussion in regard to health. When Green is careful in his articulation he speaks of *access* to health care (not health) as a primary social good: "As a result, we can expect the parties finally to opt for a principle of equal access to health care ..."[10] And in his discussion refuting the distinction Rawls makes between the goods distributed by society and those distributed by the natural lottery, Green claims that "[s]ocial decisions concerning medical care thus have a vital impact on everyone's health ..."[11] And further, Green says that "[a]ccess to health care is not only a primary social good, in Rawls's sense of the term, but possibly one of the most important such goods."[12] These statements combined indicate that Green means that access to health care has an important effect on health, and in turn, that health has an important effect on the ability to pursue various rational plans of life. Hence, the relation of health care to health for Green, seems to be a fairly straightforward one—the social distribution of health care improves the health of all citizens and thus acts as an all-purpose means by which citizens may increase their chances of successfully pursuing their respective desirable goals. Access to health care is thus a good that rational agents will want more of rather than less, in Rawlsian terms.

It should be noted, however, that in Rawls's recent work,[13] he substantially expands on the meaning of the relation of primary social goods to parties in the original position. In his revision, Rawls tends less often to characterize all the social goods as all-purpose means to rational life plans. He rather emphasizes the moral qualities of persons for the purposes of a political conception of justice. Here, he is concerned to clarify some conceptual aspects of his theory such that an inconsistency internal to his theory is removed. The inconsistency with which he is concerned involves the following: if parties to the original position are characterized as free and equal, then given the freedom equally to exercise liberties such as liberty of conscience and thought, they will naturally over time develop comprehensive religious, moral or philosophical doctrines which are not only incompatible with each other, but which are reasonable, as well. This is the fact of reasonable pluralism in a modern constitutional democracy. And because of this reasonable pluralism, agreement about the basic structure will be impossible if the principles of justice presuppose one specific comprehensive doctrine. Thus, the notion of primary social goods themselves has come under attack. If there exist reasonable, but incompatible comprehensive doctrines, then the social goods Rawls supposes people will want more of rather than less will vary along with the doctrines. And this circumstance may have a major effect on the stability of modern democracies. Thus, the question: "How is it possible that there may exist over time a stable and just society of free and equal citizens profoundly divided by reasonable religious, philosophical, and moral doctrines?"[14] The answer to this question lies in constructing a conception of justice that is independent of any particular comprehensive doctrine—that is, it is silent in respect to any of these doctrines. Instead, it tries to articulate the strictly political meanings of values, ideas and principles basic to a democracy. In this way, it hopes to gain a consensus from citizens on the political structure that, on the one hand, stands apart from their respective comprehensive doctrines, and on the other is one that they can endorse from their particular standpoints.

In order to construct such a theory, Rawls was forced into either revising some aspects of *Theory*,[15] or placing a greater emphasis on some elements. In *Theory*, Rawls most often speaks of the primary social goods as "all-purpose means" to life plans. In *Political Liberalism*, he connects the primary goods much more closely with a moral conception of persons worked up for political purposes. Here he characterizes parties to the original position as possessing two moral powers—a sense of justice and a capacity for a conception of the good—together with a correlative "highest-order" interest in developing and exercising these powers. For Rawls, "a sense of justice is the capacity to understand, to apply, and to act from the public conception of justice which characterizes the fair terms of social cooperation."[16] And a capacity for a conception of the good consists in a "capacity to form, to revise and rationally to pursue a conception of [the] good."[17] In addition, persons are attributed with a higher-order interest in a determinate conception of the good, i.e., a scheme of final ends that people pursue for their own sakes. Under this characterization of persons, the list of primary goods is to be explained "by reference to those interests."[18] That is, they are social goods that are necessary for people to act on their higher-order interests and to secure their moral powers. Thus, the primary social goods are not now to be taken merely as instrumental means to pursuing the ends comprised in comprehensive doctrines since those are ruled out of the strictly political conception of justice. Rather, they are characterized as goods which people will generally need for any particular ends *and* which protect our vital interest in acting from a sense of justice, as well as our capacity for a conception of the good. Hence, even if a social good is not one that is of use to our particular life plans, we are still able to endorse it from a political point of view because it secures what people need, *qua* citizens.

Given the preceding accounts of the role of primary goods, it might be asked whether health care is a value all rational agents would want more of rather than less, whatever their other values. In the first account (where social goods are mostly characterized as all-purpose means to particular life plans), it is certainly disputable that all would choose a principle of equal access to health care. As discussed in chapter one, there exist both religious and non-religious grounds for rejecting governmental provision of health care. To take Christian Scientists as an example, public provision of health care would force their support of a good with which they have religious disagreement. And it is precisely this sort of disagreement that threatens the stability of a society over time. The second account of the relation between primary goods and persons accounts for this objection. If the conception of justice applies only to the political arena, then a right to equal access to health care may be a good even Christian Scientists can accept because they recognize it is something which persons, as citizens, generally need to secure their highest- and higher-order interests. Otherwise put, there may be grounds, such as the principle of toleration, that allow them to affirm such a right, not because it advances their particular comprehensive doctrine, but because it is a good citizens generally need. In that case, they need not take advantage of such a right themselves, but can endorse it as part of the fair terms of social cooperation.[19] Of course, the same could be said for Rawls's earlier account of the social goods. Having equal access to health care does entail that one may take advantage of a certain good if one wants it, but it does not entail that one *must* take advantage of it. But the point is that under the new account, it is not presupposed that, say, health care is necessary for pursuing *any* determinate conception of the good. Rather the presupposition is that health care is *generally* a good necessary for people to act on their higher-order interests and their moral powers.

Green, for his part, argues that rational agents would both opt for a separate principle of access to health care, and insure that it was equally distributed to all. They would accept inequalities in less important social goods such as income and wealth as allowed by the difference principle, but maximin reasoning would not allow them to accept inequalities in access to health care. Since access to health care protects the "vital interests" of parties, they would want its distribution independent of the inequality in income allowed by the difference principle. Rational agents would choose a principle that insures "equal access to health care: each member of society, whatever his position or background, would be guaranteed an equal right to the most extensive health services the society allows."[20] However, this equal right does not signify an equal distribution, for it is not the case that everyone requires the same kind or amount of health care. Rather, "since the parties are primarily interested in securing services as they need them, equality extends only to access to the health care system."[21] Within the system, health care would be provided on the basis of need.

This leads to the second respect in which Green differs from Rawls inasmuch as he challenges the lexical priority Rawls gives to liberty over other values. In contrast to Rawls, Green argues that contracting parties would place an equal or greater value on physical well-being and security as a basis of self-esteem. Rawls claims that at a certain level of economic and social well-being, "it becomes and then remains irrational ... to acknowledge a lesser liberty for the sake of greater material means ... [because] as the general level of well-being rises ... only the less urgent wants remain to be met ..."[22] Rawls contends that less fortunate societies with less economic resources may very well find it reasonable to trade off some liberties for the sake of greater economic advantages. But once a certain level of economic efficiency is reached, individuals will have the resources to pursue their particular ends and liberties will be more valuable. And since Rawls does not allow parties the property of envy, they will not be bothered by the relative inequalities in social wealth. Thus, the ability to pursue life plans is more dependent on the various liberties, than on material means. Remembering that self-determination is bedrock to the liberal egalitarian, the priority of liberty gives individuals the self-confidence and self-respect needed to carry out their plans. Much of Rawls's argument for the priority of liberty is grounded on the psychological principle that once basic human needs such as food, warmth, and shelter are satisfied, the fundamental moral interest we have in determining our particular life plans takes precedence. "... Under favorable circumstances the fundamental interest in determining our plan of life eventually assumes a prior place."[23] And the political liberties as well as liberties such as conscience and self expression make possible the social good of self-respect, which in turn gives people a sense of the worth of their life plans.

But, argues Green, if civil and political liberties protect citizens from governmental interference in pursuing life plans, "even more apparently than governmental interference, disease and ill health interfere with our happiness and undermine our self-confidence and self-respect."[24] Hence, according to Green, Rawls should have given priority to a principle that satisfies basic human needs such as health care because of its crucial importance to life plans.

Green thus denies the legitimacy of Rawls's distinction between the social goods directly distributed by a society and natural goods only indirectly distributed by it. He rather believes that at least the natural good of health is affected by society. His claim is that modern medical technology "renders almost archaic the notion that health depends on natural contingencies ... health care ought to be considered a primary social good in [Rawls's] terms, and ought to be directly considered by a theory of justice."[25] Thus, Green argues that Rawls was mistaken in placing health care outside the scope of justice. Rather, he contends, given the conditions placed on the original position and maximin reasoning for the principles issuing from it, rational agents would not only have chosen a principle of equal access to health care, but they would have given it equal or greater lexical priority than the liberty principle.

However, Green does not insist on strict maximin reasoning in regard to health care. That is, he does not insist that society is obligated for a maximal amount of health care for the least well off. First, it is well known that maximizing the minimum amount of health care would have the effect of absorbing all the economic resources of even the richest society. In addition, according to Green, is the "common sense consideration that health is thought to be a state of mental, physical and social well-being and not merely freedom from disease."[26] On this definition of health, Green argues that a healthy existence includes freedom from economic austerity and the opportunity to exercise many human capacities which, in turn, requires expenditure of public resources. It is expenditures such as research for improved medical technology which Green says will conflict with health care spending, and which will lead maximin reasoners to accept less than the "best possible" health care. He thus argues for equal access to a decent minimum of health care at the beginning stages of economic development. The decent minimum would include basic preventive and therapeutic services. However, at later stages of economic development he suggests that more intensive preventive programs, more sophisticated therapies, and more esoteric medical research should be included because "maximin reasoning counsels protecting oneself as much as possible against ill health."[27]

Green further suggests that at this later stage of development real members of actual societies might decide to distribute health care through free market mechanisms because those will allow individuals to establish priorities between health care and other goods and might improve the quality and efficiency of the health care system. However, in order to retain the goal of equal access to health care, progressive rates on services may need to be introduced. Here, it might be remarked that a social guarantee to a decent minimum of health care combined with a free market mechanism of distribution (using the device of progressive rates), will allow a two-tiered system of health care delivery. Those at the bottom of society will still not be able to afford the more esoteric health care services that the better off can. However, this circumstance, by itself, is not objectionable on a Rawlsian account of justice since he allows inequalities so long as they benefit all. If health care is distributed by free market mechanisms and if, in fact, that mechanism improves the quality and efficiency of health care for all, then the inequalities should be permissible. The resulting configuration would be, then, equal access to a decent minimum of health care, with those at intermediate and upper levels of wealth being able to afford progressively more esoteric or sophisticated health care.

Problems With Green's Proposal

We should remember that Rawls argues for the priority of the equal liberty principle for several reasons. First, it seems to him that civil and political liberties are fundamental values of liberal democracies. But second, they are extremely important means to individual life plans, the pursuit of which is foundational to liberal egalitarianism as well as central to the exercise of the moral powers. And finally, Rawls is attempting to systematize moral intuitions basic to liberal democracies. That is, liberal intuitions about the distribution of freedoms, opportunities and income and wealth frequently come into conflict when we attempt to apply them to actual societies. Since Rawls believes that civil and political liberties possess both value in themselves and are instrumental means to the most important social goods, he gives them lexical priority over the other social goods. Thus, when conflicts arise between the liberties and other goods, his theory supplies us with a rationale for preferring liberty over opportunity and opportunity over income and wealth.

Moreover, it is Rawls's claim that once we start importing specified principles of justice into a theoretical structure, we increase the risk of conflicting principles. In that event, we simply have no way to weigh their moral importance. For example, how do we weigh the moral importance of providing health care against the value of providing protection from both internal and external harms if both are valued equally among the primary social goods?

However, Green claims that conflicts between the liberty principle and a health care principle are rare. Or more precisely, he claims that "conflicts between the civil liberties and health care are not so common as to force a relative evaluation of the two."[28] Green seems to be suggesting two things here. First, he seems to be suggesting that the rights associated with the liberties (e.g., the right to equal protection under the law) rarely would conflict with a right to equal access to health care. And second, since these rights rarely conflict, we need not bother evaluating their importance against each other to persons regarded as free and equal. If, in fact, it is the case that these rights rarely conflict, then Green may be correct that we need not bother evaluating their relative importance.

Yet, a right to equal access to health care may quite easily come into conflict with the liberties, if not directly, at least where funding for these rights is concerned. For example, one of the more forceful objections to the death penalty is that it's unevenly distributed, with the poor and racial minorities receiving the death penalty more frequently than rich, white individuals.[29] This circumstance is largely the result of the disadvantaged's inability to afford better legal defense. Rather, they are assigned public defenders who are inexperienced in the practice of law, and who are extremely overburdened by their case loads. (In fact, the justice system is now so overloaded that a new term has been coined: "fast-food justice.") One way to reduce this problem is to pour more money into the justice system so that defendants have more equal representation. But if we follow Green's line of thinking (where access to health care is as important as equal protection under the law), it will be difficult to tell which right has funding priority. So it seems we do, after all, need to evaluate the relative importance of a right to health care against the rights associated with the civil liberties if they are to be given equal priority as Green claims in the determination of the basic structure of society. But how this is to be accomplished on Green's extension of Rawls's contract theory is unclear.

How might we work out the ranking of health care in which conflicts do not arise? We can begin by giving the equal access to health care principle lexical priority over the equal liberties principle. And here I am assuming that entailed by the lexical priority of the principles and the satisfaction of the first before the satisfaction of the second in actual societies not only must the rights be in place, but at least partial funding must be set aside, as well.[30] If we give lexical priority to the health care principle, then in order to fit it into Rawls's theory, it would have to be satisfied before the liberty principle.[31] This would mean that before rights such as a right to equal protection under the law are satisfied, a right to health care must be stabilized. It would also mean that political liberties, religious liberty and free expression would be curtailed or limited if that would increase general access to health care. For example, before the legal apparatus required for equal protection is established and funded, medical facilities and funding would need to be set up. Is this arrangement plausible? If health care gains its significance because of its great instrumental value in protecting plans of life, then what distinguishes it as more important than a right to equal protection under the law? It seems that both equally play pivotal roles in that regard.

Thus, priority of the equal health care principle over the equal liberties principle seems implausible.

This leaves us with a second option of inserting the health care principle between the liberties principle and the fair equality of opportunity principle. Here the equal liberties principle will retain its priority, but equal opportunity will be moved down a notch in its competition for social resources. Rawls rarely comments on the practical implications of his principles. But he makes an exception in the case of opportunity, for he allows that public resources may be required to make this principle a reality as opposed to a merely formal right. In order to mitigate the effects of social standing, public funding for educational programs such as Headstart may be required.[32] Education, as we all know, requires large public expenditures, yet it seems crucial to securing equal chances to "enjoy the culture of [a] society and to take part in its affairs, and ... to provide for each individual a secure sense of his own worth."[33] Again, this solution to the priority problem seems implausible because funding for health care will take priority over funding for opportunity. And not only Rawls, but most liberal theorists make a general appeal to the importance of education in protecting equal opportunity because of the latter's contribution to life plans.

But if health care is as important to life plans as it intuitively seems to be, then Rawls's theory must somehow accommodate our health care concerns, for at rock bottom he justifies all his principles by appeal to their contribution to individual life plans. It is, as Green points out, something no rational agent in an initial situation of equality would agree to do without. And Rawls, himself, is not unaware of the seriousness of the problem of health care. He concedes that using his original notion of primary social goods works only when we "assume that all citizens have physical and psychological capacities within a certain normal range."[34] He continues that if a solution can be worked out for the normal health and medical needs of citizens "at the legislative stage in the light of existing social conditions, then it may be possible to extend it to people who have special needs ... [but] if it cannot be worked out ... the idea of primary goods may have to be abandoned."[35] However, it is unclear how the notion of primary goods can be abandoned without abandoning the core of Rawls's theory, for the principles which he argues will issue from the original position are to be assessed in terms of how well they secure the social primary goods.

There remain four possibilities for incorporating health care into the basic formulation.

First, so long as it is consistent with the two main principles, we might locate a principle of health care after the second principle. This, in effect, is what Rawls does with the principle of efficiency. However, given the structure and intent of Rawls's theory, this, too, seems implausible. If we assume that a right to health care is spelled out in terms of an *equal* access to health care services, then this right would have to fall in the lexical ordering *prior* to the difference principle because the difference principle acts to compensate for any remaining inequalities after the equal liberties and opportunity principles have been satisfied.

We might try inserting it as a separate section in the second principle. Then the second principle might have a lexical ordering in which income inequalities are compensated after equal liberties, opportunities and access to health care have been satisfied. However, I do not see how this ordering could escape the objection that educational and health care benefits may compete for the same monies and for the same reason: that both are essential to life plans. Thus, which principle—opportunity or health care—should be lexically prior is indeterminate because they both serve the same purpose on this account. Otherwise put, it's unclear to what legislators could appeal to make funding decisions in real time that gives priority to funding health care over education, or education over funding.

The third possibility involves the difference principle. It could be the case that health care costs which reduce income below a level that makes it impossible for people, e.g., to pursue their own conceptions of the good would be compensated by health care benefits. This is precisely the sort of compensation with which the difference principle is designed to deal. In other words, even though individuals are disadvantaged by their natural circumstances, they are still entitled to the social goods, including the wherewithal to pursue their reasonable life plans, distributed by society. We could thus attempt to derive a right to health care from the difference principle. But then the right cannot be construed solely in terms of an *equal* right of access, for only the most disadvantaged in society will have a social guarantee to health care benefits. Those whose ability to pursue life plans is unaffected by health care costs would not qualify for compensation. At most, on this formulation, health care benefits can play only a compensatory role on Rawls's theory. For instance, money might be provided by government to compensate health care providers such that the least well off do not fall below a decent income level. It might be noted in this regard that the only thing that distinguishes this system from the one presently existing in the US is that one must fall below the poverty level *first* before one is eligible for Medicaid; while on the difference principle, one would be *prevented* from falling below the poverty level.

There are thus at least three problems on Green's proposal for extending Rawls's theory to health care. None of the possible orderings of an equal access to health care explain why it might be more fundamental to pursuing life plans than either the basic liberties or opportunity principles. And second, if the proposed health care principle is given equal status to the opportunity principle, then conflicts over priority in funding are almost sure to arise in real time. And finally, if the health care principle is somehow associated with the difference principle, then access to health care will not be equal—it will rather be more like the system we already have. Thus introducing a separate principle for health care into the Rawlsian scheme as Green proposes turns out to be extremely difficult without reworking Rawls's whole schema.

There remains one possibility: that a principle of health care can be derived from the fair equality of opportunity principle in Rawls's basic formulation. This is the project that Norman Daniels has set for himself and with which I deal in the next chapter.

CHAPTER 3

NORMAN DANIELS'S EXTENSION OF RAWLS'S THEORY

We saw the difficulties in the last chapter with attempting to introduce a separate, fundamental principle into a Rawlsian scheme of justice. But there are two problems, as I see it. First, none of the possible orderings of an equal access to health care principle explains its fundamental importance to life plans over the two principles of justice set out by Rawls. This inability is the priority problem: there seems to be no plausible explanation why access to health care is more fundamental than liberties or opportunities in pursuing life plans. One reason it may be difficult to explain is simply that health care is not more fundamental than liberty and opportunity. A second reason may be that even if health care is fundamental, it is extremely difficult to add elements to Rawls's theory without at the same time disturbing its equilibrium. The theory is so finely tuned that adding or subtracting anything tends to throw the whole system of justice off kilter. That is, the lexical priority of values in Rawls's theory means that if A has priority over B, then A cannot be sacrificed, traded or limited in order to secure B. Thus if liberty has priority over health care, then liberty cannot be limited to increase access to health care. But since Green cannot offer us a reasonable explanation for the priority of health care, there remains a gap in explaining why it is a social responsibility and not simply a good to be governed by the free market. Hence, on Rawls's theory, the priority problem actually turns out to be a problem for the macroallocation of social goods not governed by the two principles of justice for which he argues. If no reasonable explanation is offered concerning the priority of, e.g., the good of health care, then attempting to fit it into a Rawlsian scheme of justice will fail. And if it fails, then we have no principled way to assign weight to a right to health care against a right to liberties and opportunities. And if we cannot weigh it, then the design of institutions that would embody such a right becomes extremely difficult.

The second problem arises from the first. We have not been convinced that health care is of equal or greater importance than liberty and opportunity in the pursuit of life plans, and yet we intuitively see a connection between health care and our success in life. Hence, not only do we not know how to rank its importance, but even if we somehow incorporated it into Rawls's theory, we do not know how to ration the various kinds and amounts of health care within a system. This is a problem of indeterminacy in application. Let me explain. We might think that the whole of Rawls's theory taken together, implies a social obligation to provide access to health care.[1] Yet the design of actual institutions requires not only some purchase on how to prioritize funding among social goods, but also how to ration the funding within any particular institution, e.g., the institution of health care, itself. Even if we could somehow figure out the macroallocation (priority between various social goods), we do not have a principled way to figure out the microallocations (rationing of health care within the health care system when resources are limited). The problem is this: we have yet to set up a fair procedure to decide among various health-care goods that might obligate society as opposed to health-care goods that are outside the scope of social obligations. We thus have two separate problems: the priority among different social goods at the macro level, and the indeterminacy in application (the micro level), assuming that priorities could be arranged.

On Rawls's theory, we might suppose this second problem has a solution by taking seriously his idea that inequalities are permissible so long as they benefit the least well off. But here again, it's unclear how to understand this. Does it mean that health care costs that reduce one's income below legitimate expectations[2] ought to be compensated by the difference principle? Or does it mean that those who are least well off in respect to health (despite their income level), should be provided health care? If we understand "least well off" in the first sense, then the right to health care will not be an equal one. If we understand "least well off" in the second sense, to how much and what kinds of health care are those individuals entitled, the maximal amount? That seems implausible given the costs it would impose on the more healthy. But giving no priority to the least healthy and least able to provide for themselves seems implausible as well, for what seems to be crucially involved in a right to health care is to insure that those in great need are not left to fend for themselves when they cannot meet their own needs. This means that the term "worst off" needs to be spelled out for a system of health care delivery. "Worst off" might mean both the worst off in terms of financial arrangements and the worst off in terms of health. Hence, society would have an obligation only for the poorest and least healthy. This account of our obligation seems unsatisfactory, however, for if there are reasons that justify providing health care for only the poorest and the least healthy—those with extreme needs—would not those reasons also suffice for ordinary care? That is, if the goods of society are to be distributed fairly, why would a society agree to spend excessive resources on those with extreme needs, but not meet the ordinary needs of its citizens?

Norman Daniels has attempted to deal with both the macro and the microallocation problems just discussed (the priority of a social obligation to provide health care and the attempt to provide determinate guidelines for allocation within the health care system).[3] He begins with the questions, Why is health care special? What does it do for us that might give it a special moral importance? His analysis of health care ultimately connects it to the idea of social justice.

The Priority of Health Care

Daniels first notes that health care serves many functions, some of which are more urgent or important than others. Health care can extend or save lives, and it can improve the quality of life in various ways. For instance, it generally has the ability to reduce suffering and maintain or restore people to normal (or more normal) functioning. However, it also has the ability to improve appearances through cosmetic treatments or extend life beyond a point where it is reasonable to say that quality of life is maintained. It is precisely because health care has the ability to serve functions such as these last two, that Daniels wants to distinguish those kinds of health care for which society is obligated and those for which it is not. One way of doing this is by making a distinction between needs and preferences.

This distinction is familiar to anyone with knowledge of a consequentialist approach to moral theory in contrast to a deontological approach. Utilitarianism, one form of consequentialism, takes as its basic principle either promoting the greatest happiness of all those affected by an action or policy, or the greatest satisfaction of preferences by all those affected. This principle has led to several objections, one of which is that those with extravagant tastes will require more in the way of goods to make them happy than those with more modest tastes. In this circumstance, so the objection runs, those with more modest tastes will be unfairly forced to make sacrifices for the benefit of those with expensive tastes. This problem arises for utilitarianism because it does not place an independent value on just distributions of goods.

However, Daniels has adopted a deontological view just because he believes that justice in the distribution of goods ought to have a value independent of promoting happiness or satisfaction of preferences. We can understand this more clearly by setting it in a context. Suppose that one individual would be content only if he were provided the most extensive cosmetic surgery made available by advanced technology. A second individual may be content to get a flu shot once a year. If health care were a social obligation justified by the principle of utility, then the second individual's interests may be sacrificed (even if she is content with only a flu shot) because large amounts of social resources will be taken up in satisfying the preferences of the first. But this seems to be an unfair distribution of social resources, quite independently of how the second individual feels about her treatment. Hence, Daniels claims that for the purposes of social justice, there needs to be a way to separate the things people need to pursue their lives from the things people would like. Put another way, Daniels adopts a Rawlsian idea concerning social justice: society is responsible for a just framework of liberties and opportunities within which individuals can pursue life plans, but individuals within that society are assumed the ability to regulate their preferences in line with what they can legitimately expect given that framework. Daniels (as well as Rawls) thus considers a limited number of social goods as necessary means to individual life plans. These necessary means, then, are a special category of needs required by social justice.

The way in which Daniels separates out citizens' needs from preferences is by noticing two central properties needs possess. They are objectively ascribable and objectively important. Objectively ascribable needs are ones we can attribute to someone simply in virtue of her being a member of a species. Hence, independently of one's own preferences, these needs are things members of a species require throughout their entire lives, but exclude things required for any particular 'contingent projects' one may have. Objectively ascribable, or course-of-life, needs include "food, shelter, clothing, exercise, rest, companionship, a mate (in one's prime), and so on ... a deficiency with respect to any of these needs endangers the normal functioning of the subject of need *considered as a member of a natural species*."[4] Or, as McCloskey puts it, needs "relate to what it would be detrimental to us to lack, where the detrimental is explained by reference to our natures as men and specific persons."[5] Using these references to define the general sorts of needs that are objectively ascribable and important, Daniels claims that given an "appropriate notion of species-typical functioning" health care needs are objectively ascribable.

Objectively important needs, according to Daniels, are important because they are either the kinds of goods typically thought to be a requirement of justice, or because there is a relationship between them and the "other, general kinds of social goods which are the subject matter of general theories of distributive justice."[6] These sorts of goods, Daniels argues, have a weightier moral claim than mere personal preferences. One such good is opportunity, or as Daniels puts it, a "range of opportunity open to the individual in which he may construct his 'plan of life' or 'conception of the good.'"[7] So if people have a pressing interest in "preserving the opportunity to revise their conceptions of the good through time, then they will have a pressing interest in maintaining normal species functioning by establishing institutions, such as health-care systems, which do just that."[8] The kinds of needs picked out by reference to normal species functioning, then, are objectively important because they "meet this fundamental interest persons have in maintaining a normal range of opportunities."[9] Hence, a scale of goods can be constructed that separates social obligations from individual preferences. Since health care needs, according to Daniels, are both objectively ascribable and objectively important (they protect one sort of goods with which distributive justice is concerned), they meet the requirements of a social obligation.

Daniels, however, does not insist as Green has done, that health care is a primary social good which ought to be covered by its own separate principle. The chief reason he does not is precisely the problem that Green encounters: once we include health care as a distinct social good and introduce a separate principle governing it, we run into the problem of weighing it against "opportunity, income, powers and other social goods."[10] So for Daniels, while health care needs are not directly a part of a just framework, they are nonetheless 'special,' or important, in the sense that they help protect the normal range of opportunities reasonable persons may expect to pursue in a given society.

It is worthwhile to recall, here, the liberal egalitarian basis of Rawls's and Daniels's theories. Fundamental to this type of theory is the idea that individual lives go best when they are determined from the 'inside.' Individuals are not only happier when their lives are self-determined, but they are shown the respect they deserve as rational, autonomous agents when interference in their self-chosen plans is held to a minimum. This underlying basis of egalitarianism explains the importance we give to the values of liberty and equality. If one starts from the fairly uncontroversial assumption that individuals are moral equals, one need not carry that assumption to the absurd conclusion that individuals are equals in every sense. Obviously people have different abilities, skills, and talents as well as belonging to different social classes. Of course, belonging to different social classes is often a result of possessing different abilities and so on. It seems to be the case that those possessing greater abilities often occupy more socially desirable positions. However, it is not always the case: some are held back merely because of socially erected obstacles. But if we take seriously the idea of moral equality, then socially erected obstacles are unjust, according to Rawls and Daniels. Justice thus requires that those having roughly equal skills and talents are guaranteed an equal opportunity in the competition for desirable positions. It is from this perspective that Daniels claims people have a fundamental interest in preserving their share of the range of opportunity in which they may conceive and revise their life plans consistent with the features found in their society: the level of economic and technological development, its historical development and the conception of justice regulating its basic institutions. These features, argues Daniels, determine the normal opportunity range within any given society, and properties possessed by individuals determine their share of that opportunity range when they are functioning normally. However, as

Daniels notes, disease and disability shrink an individual's share of the normal opportunity range from what is fair.

The result of this explanation of citizens' needs is a list of primary social goods for which society is responsible and those are distinct from the preferences for which individuals are responsible. Although health care, itself, is not a primary social good, it is associated with one: namely, equal opportunity, and it is so, for Daniels, because of its strategic importance in protecting opportunities. This move allows Daniels to assign some priority to a right to health care indirectly without at the same time giving rise to conflicting claims concerning priority between liberty and equality rights.[11] In turn, this associative priority offers some guidelines for the macroallocation of health care. The lexical priority of liberty will require its satisfaction before steps are taken to insure equal opportunity. But once liberty rights are satisfied, steps to satisfy equality of opportunity must be taken.

The Moral Justification of a Right to Health Care

Daniels's notion that health care protects equal opportunity has so far been simply a description. But since a social obligation to provide health care depends crucially on the idea of opportunity, something needs to be said about how we are to understand it and whether some understanding of it justifies a social obligation to provide health care.

There are strong disagreements about what equality of opportunity requires, or even means. The prevailing justification for economic inequalities is that they are morally acceptable provided there was fair competition among the contenders in the awarding of offices and positions. Where conservatives and liberals part ways is over the meaning of "fair competition." The conservative adopts the view that differences in economic status are morally acceptable so long as they were the result of native skills and talents, and the choices people have made in developing them. Unequal economic distributions are unfair, however, if the competition for advantageous positions is biased by differences which are irrelevant to the competition. Class, race, age, and sex are the usual examples of irrelevant discriminations in awarding most positions. The key idea behind this version of equality of opportunity is that competitions are unfair when the criteria for hiring or awarding positions are irrelevant to whether or not the task can be accomplished. It seems to follow, then, that competitions are fair when the criterion is simply that individuals can accomplish a task because of their choices and efforts in developing whatever natural talents and skills they happen to have.

This interpretation of fair competition (or equal opportunity) is what Daniels calls the 'negative interpretation,' and what Rawls has called 'formal equality of opportunity.' At most, formal equality of opportunity acts as a negative constraint on hiring practices. For instance, it prohibits anti-black or sexist hiring laws or practices. Thus, the conservative will say that if laws exist which prohibit discrimination based on class, sex, age, race or ethnicity, then the competition was fair as are the economic inequalities that attach to them. On the conservative view, then, society is not obligated to provide extra means for those in socially disadvantaging circumstances, the assumption being that individuals can bootstrap themselves out of those conditions.

However, the Rawlsian interpretation of fair competition digs deeper into background conditions. It says that prohibiting discrimination based on irrelevant characteristics does not go far enough, for it does not compensate for inequalities due to social class or family upbringing. Rawls, along with Daniels, argues that formal equality of opportunity does not amount to actual equality because it does not correct for negative influences affecting people's ability to compete for positions. Some have been luckier in their place in the social lottery, yet none strictly deserve the advantages conferred by their place. An individual may have been born into a privileged family and received greater educational benefits which, strictly speaking, she has not earned, i.e., these are circumstances for which she is not responsible. Both Rawls and Daniels argue that though the social lottery is arbitrary, justice can do better. They mean by this that a just basic structure of society should not allow the arbitrariness of the social lottery to determine socially advantageous distributions of jobs and positions. On this positive view of equality of opportunity, there exists a social obligation to correct for circumstances that put people at a disadvantage in the competition for desirable positions. This positive conception of equality of opportunity is what Rawls call 'fair equality of opportunity.' On this conception, there may very well exist a social obligation to provide additional educational benefits such as Headstart for children from impoverished families.

Rawls further argues that once we are bothered by socially disadvantaging circumstances in the competition for jobs and positions, we should be bothered by naturally occurring disadvantages, as well. Here, Rawls continues making a distinction between the choices for which we are responsible and circumstances for which we are not. Just as people do not deserve their place in the social lottery, they do not deserve their advantaging talents and skills. However, Rawls does not propose that we compensate for natural disadvantages in the same way as the fair equality of opportunity principle requires for social disadvantages. Rather, he says we are led to the so-called difference principle that is designed to insure that the worst off in society are not disadvantaged in the distribution of social goods. Of course, the difference principle does not remove all disadvantages, but it does render inequalities acceptable. Further, they will be entitled to equal liberties and opportunities and by the difference principle, at least be assured of an income that allows them to pursue reasonable life plans. But unlike the fair equality of opportunity principle that may require extra educational benefits for the disadvantaged, Rawls does not offer any additional compensation for naturally occurring disadvantages such as ill health except through the difference principle.

One reason Rawls does not require direct compensation for natural disadvantages in the same way as social disadvantages is that his theory is an idealizing one. It applies to individuals who are "normal, active, and fully cooperating members of society over the course of a complete life."[12] Working out a theory of justice is difficult enough without attempting to equalize the variables in peoples' talents, skills and physical capabilities (even if that were possible). So Rawls's hope is that once the idealized, or easy, case for a theory of justice is worked out, it can be modified or extended for the hard cases.

We might suppose that Rawls's so-called difference principle would be able to accommodate the hard cases. Basically, its intention is to insure a claim to compensation by those who are either socially or naturally disadvantaged such that their bundle of primary social goods is not arbitrarily diminished because of their circumstances. However, two aspects of Rawls's theory work against the difference principle as an adequate safe-guard for hard cases such as ill health. First, as already mentioned, it fails to include those who have medical needs. And second, the difference principle measures the well being of individuals against income and wealth rather than physical health. So, if two people were equally well-off, but one had greater health-care costs, that difference would not be compensated by the difference principle. Thus, the costs of ill health not only are not compensated, but we can suppose that the ability to lead a successful life is also compromised.[13] So, indeed, Rawls must rely on an extension or a modification of his theory to cover cases such as ill health.

This is precisely what Daniels attempts to do. He adopts the fair equality of opportunity principle, but points out that the idealizing conditions set out by Rawls's theory do not make allowances for people with diseases or disabilities. Hence, he broadens the fair equality of opportunity principle to include not just social disadvantages, but natural disadvantages as well. Further, Daniels notes that once we drop the idealizing conditions and allow for natural disadvantages, and if we measure fair shares of primary goods by reference to income and wealth, we will find that those with equal indices will not be equally well-off. Once health-care costs are subtracted from their incomes, those individuals would not have equal indices provided that the index took into account health-care costs (but the index does not take those costs into account on Rawls's formulation). Thus, individuals, who through no fault of their own are beset by disease and disability, will typically have greater health care expenses that will reduce their incomes below what they might legitimately expect. In that case, they may not have the resources to pursue plans of life that would otherwise be reasonable for them.

In addition, our social circumstances affect our state of health—it is well known that people with little or no disposable income and no health insurance, wait longer to see a physician when they are ill. As a result, their physical health suffers. Under non-ideal conditions, then, the distinction that Rawls has made between choices for which one is responsible and circumstances for which one is not responsible and which influence ability to compete for positions, collapses. Our social circumstances may be determined not so much by our choices as by undeserved influences such as disease and disability. Hence, according to Daniels, the natural lottery can no more be ignored than the social lottery. Daniels thus concludes that under non-ideal conditions, the distinction Rawls has made between choices and circumstances ought to be extended to natural disadvantages. Daniels thus offers a conditional justification for health care as a social obligation:

> Health-care institutions should be among those governed by a principle of fair equality of opportunity, provided two conditions obtain: (1) an acceptable general theory of justice includes a principle which requires basic institutions to guarantee fair equality of opportunity, and (2) the fair equality of opportunity principle acts as a constraint on permissible economic inequalities.[14]

The central, moral importance of health care, then, is its effect on people's ability to conceive, pursue and revise life plans which are both satisfying and reasonable were it not for impairments of normal species functioning affecting their share of the normal opportunity range. The idea is that impairment of normal functioning through disease and disability reduces an individual's fair share of the opportunity range from what she otherwise could expect given her natural talents and preferences, thus putting her at a disadvantage in pursuing her determinate goals. Thus, a social obligation to provide health care is morally justified because of its contribution to protecting fair equality of opportunity. If justice requires fair equality of opportunity, then it also requires access to health care.

Something is missing, however, from this account of the relation between social justice and health care. Rawls's fair equality of opportunity principle is chiefly concerned with how the distribution of offices and positions affects life plans. Daniels argues that this is a narrow interpretation of fair equality of opportunity. He continues by pointing out that people have age-appropriate conceptions of the good throughout a lifetime.

> Life plans clearly have stages, which reflect important divisions in the life cycle ... it is easy to observe that lives have phases in which different tasks are central: nurturing and training in childhood and youth, pursuit of career and family in adult years, and the completion of life projects in later years.[15]

Given that individuals have plans throughout their lives, the narrower interpretation of fair equality of opportunity would result in a morally objectionable distribution of health care—one that is age-biased; for it makes reference to life plans in terms of careers and positions in public life, rather than in terms of retirement from public life. Daniels thus argues that even though the elderly have greater health care needs, prudent health care planners would adopt a system of health care that protects normal species functioning at all stages of life. He adopts Rawls's strategy in arguing for an 'age-relative opportunity range' by imposing a suitably thinned veil of ignorance. Prudent planners, in deciding on principles to govern their social cooperation, would be ignorant of their age, health status, genetic history or particular conceptions of the good. But they would have access to other important facts about their society that bear on health and disease. And they would also recognize that our plans change with the stages in our lives. Rawls's fair equality of opportunity might be able to accommodate the first two stages, but clearly the third stage requires the broader principle of equal opportunity. Thus, "Prudent deliberators, appropriately constrained, would seek a health care and long-term-care system that protected their normal opportunity range at each stage of their lives."[16] The principle with which Daniels started has now been modified considerably to include both natural disadvantages and life plans understood in a less traditional way: they are not just to be understood in terms of careers, but the plans we have over a complete lifetime.

Are these modifications reasonable? Taking them separately, the first seems *prima facie* reasonable once we drop Rawls's idealizing conditions. The affect of ill health on life plans is obvious, and if we follow that line of thinking, the effect of health care on ill health seems equally obvious in most cases. In a majority of cases, health care will protect an individual's share of the opportunity range. If health care increases an individual's chances of pursuing life plans and if equal opportunity is fundamental to a general theory of distributive justice, then health care seems to be a social obligation.

The second modification seems equally reasonable once we drop the idealizing conditions to accommodate both the facts of ill health and increased life expectancies. People, in fact, do make plans for their retirements that increasingly may take up a full 20-30% of their entire lives. If life plans retain their importance upon retirement, then it seems "prudent planners" would indeed choose a health care plan that protected them at each stage of their lives. Hence, both of these modifications taken separately seem reasonable.

I started this chapter, however, by noting that two general problems exist concerning access to health care. The first is the priority problem and it concerns a reasonable explanation as to the priority of different social goods. Daniels offers what seems to me to be a reasonable explanation of the priority of health care. On his account, we are not asked to accept the proposition that a right to health care is more fundamental than liberty, nor are we asked to somehow work out the priority of such a right against another fundamental right, that of opportunity. Thus, assignment of the macroallocation of health care services by its lexical priority does not give rise to confusion. That is to say, it does not tend to throw Rawls's system of justice into disequilibrium. And all that is required of us is accepting the relation between health care and equal opportunity that seems, in my opinion, a reasonable proposition.

However, a *theory* of just health care must be able to do more than give us a moral justification of access to health care for which the priority of goods has a plausible explanation. Given the assumption that resources are limited, it also must provide guidelines for the microallocation of health care services within that system if it is to be useful in guiding public policy. This is the subject to which I now turn.

The Microallocation of Health Care Services

I have several times mentioned the idea of normal species functioning. For Daniels, the task of defining normal species functioning lies with the biomedical sciences that draws on "a theoretical account of the design of the organism."[17] The organism here, of course, is homo sapiens. As such, an account must include not only our strictly biological functions, but those functions as they relate to us as social animals. Hence, the definition must account for more than just cellular functions, more than just an ability to digest food or procreate, and so on. It must also be capable of characterizing the underlying biological structures that make possible our ability to communicate, or to acquire knowledge, or to cooperate with each other under various circumstances. In addition, Daniels assumes that, at least in the future, the biomedical model of species functioning can explain psychopathology, i.e., the physiological functions that affect our ability to be social creatures. He thus assumes that even if we do not yet have a developed account of mental disease, its underlying cause is biological and thus generates a health care need.[18]

What counts for health on this model, then, is the absence of dysfunctional biological systems which negatively affect our ability to digest, procreate, maintain homeostasis, and so on, *and* our ability to function socially. Hence, diseases on this account, are "*deviations from the natural functional organization of a typical member of a species.*"[19] Having thus given us a justification for the macroallocation of health care, Daniels now sets out to specify the kinds of health care for which society is obligated. Otherwise put, the microallocation of health care needs is set by two criteria: defining disease and noting the effect disease has on the normal opportunity range of individuals.

The biomedical model of disease may seem to be a rather narrow one, for it takes health care services as 'fixed primarily by nature', and does not expand the notion of health to some broader notion of well-being as the World Health Organization does,[20] and which is basically the definition of health that Ronald Green adopts: "health is thought to be a state of mental, physical and social well-being and not merely freedom from disease."[21] However, Daniels says that "health is not happiness and confusing the two over-medicalizes social philosophy."[22] Presumably, what Daniels means here is that one may be happy without being healthy, or healthy without being happy, and at any rate, justice in the distribution of goods concerns the right (or the means) to pursue happiness, but does not guarantee happiness, itself.

With respect to the second criterion (the effect disease has on the normal opportunity range), Daniels has already argued that health care services ought to be governed by a broadened fair equality of opportunity principle. The notion of a normal opportunity range appears in this context. Recall that given certain features of society, there exists some normal opportunity range in which people may pursue their own ends. Further, within that range, individual shares are determined by their native skills and talents. But as Daniels points out, "impairment of normal functioning through disease and disability restricts an individual's opportunity *relative to that portion of the normal range his skills and talents would have made available to him were he healthy.*"[23] Thus, the kind of health care for which society is obliged reaches only so far as disease and disability reduce an individual's fair share of the opportunity range.

We might think, however, that since Daniels has broadened the fair equality of opportunity principle to include life plans rather than the narrower notion of opportunity which limits it to the pursuit of careers, that the kinds of health care obligating society may be quite broad indeed. It seems quite fair to ask whether society is duty-bound to provide services that support *any* plan of life. Obviously, Daniels has limited health care obligations by reference to the biological model. But he has also broadened the scope of health care access by his moral justification of a right to such access. The short answer to the question is: it is unclear. Let me explain.

First, Daniels does not think that society necessarily has an obligation to provide health care that will return individuals to a plan of life they have already chosen should disease or disability strike. This is what he calls one's *effective* opportunity—the opportunity, or plan of life, which an individual has actually chosen. Rather, there exists some *range* of opportunity for each individual that is determined by both her talents and skills *and* the general conditions of her society. Within that range, there may be several appropriate plans of life. When disease or disability shrink that range from what is fair, then the broadened principle of fair equality of opportunity says that the kinds of health care services obligating society are those that preserve at least some portion of an individual's share. Society is not obligated to return an individual to her former life plan, but merely to some portion of her range. And, keeping in mind that disease is defined as departures from normal species functioning, health care services obligating society are only those that maintain normal functioning. Thus, if an individual's plan of life requires health services above and beyond normal functioning *and* some portion of her range of opportunity is intact, then society is not obligated for those needs.

A simple example might help. We might suppose a woman with the requisite skills and talents to pursue various life plans: a traditional wife and mother, an artist who combines her artistic talents with mothering, and someone who is capable of, and wants to pursue only a career. Within this last group, there exist several options, but only one of which she really wants: she wants to be an exotic dancer. She has the skills and talents for this career, but she does not have the physical endowment (large breasts) that would make her competitive. I use this example because Daniels, himself, makes a distinction between reconstructive surgery for women who have suffered breast cancer and women who want mammoplasty for purely cosmetic reasons.[24] Reconstructive surgery, Daniels insists, returns the cancer patient to some level of normal functioning (a requirement of justice), but since small breast size is not a disease, society is not obligated by justice to improve our woman's chances to compete at least in this particular career.

In other words, Daniels restricts a social obligation to provide health care in two ways. First, by defining disease by reference to a biomedical model so that not all available health care services oblige society; only departures from normal species functioning do. And second, by insisting that personal preferences in the choice of life plans do not determine the kinds of health care for which society is obligated. Rather, the range of opportunity open to an individual should not be shrunk from what is fair. Hence, society is not obligated to improve an individual's prospects for a particular life plan so long as some portion of her range is still open to her. Daniels thus hopes to maintain the distinction between personal preferences and objectively important needs by appealing to the notion of a normal opportunity range, in light of which some plans of life are reasonable and some are not.

However, we can still ask the obvious, What is a fair portion of an individual's opportunity range? Or better, what is a *reasonable* life plan that, in turn, obligates society? Answer: that portion which would be open to the individual were it not for disease and disability, but not necessarily anything which an individual might prefer. In other words, plans of life which would be reasonable to choose are those constituted by (1) the conditions of society, (2) individual skills, talents and natural attributes, and (3) which would constitute over the long run the good life for an agent. Thus, our would-be exotic dancer has chosen an unreasonable life plan because while she possesses the skills and talents necessary for the job, she lacks a crucial natural attribute which is at the same time, not a disease or disability. This conclusion indicates that not *any* plan of life is supported by Daniels's account, only reasonable ones, where the reasonable is explained by reference to a constellation of skills, talents, natural attributes and social conditions and which at the same time blocks personal preferences.

What remains unexplained in this account, is the actual differences between the reasonable and personal preferences as the breast reconstruction example shows. If the reason Daniels believes that the cancer patient is due reconstructive surgery is because it returns her to normal functioning, how are we to understand this? Roughly, there seem to be two functions of the breast. The first is a natural function: to nourish the young. The second is a social construct: making women more sexually attractive to men. Reconstructive surgery to the mastectomy patient will not return the normal functioning of the breast (assuming the mastectomy is radical). However, it might return the second (social construct) function. But this is precisely the reason the exotic dancer wants breast enhancement. What makes this doubly confusing is that in either case, the idea of a life plan enters the picture. Why is the mastectomy patient's life plan more reasonable than the exotic dancer's? It cannot be because the first one's goal is more worthy (even if some think it is), because the worthiness of a goal is irrelevant from the perspective of liberal egalitarianism. This kind of theory explicitly refrains from making judgments on the worth of a life plan, but rather places value on the framework of rights and opportunities which enable people to pursue plans of their *own* choosing whatever they may be, so long as they do not violate the principles of justice. The value of living one's life from the inside, then, is the emphasis, not the worth of any particular plan. This analysis suggests that Daniels, if he is to be consistent, must accept breast enhancement as part of a package of health care needs provided by society, or he must put constraints on treatments such as reconstructive surgery if they do not significantly affect an individual's normal share of the opportunity range.

This conclusion implies two things: First, once a range of opportunity is introduced, it's extremely difficult to keep a bright-line distinction between personal preferences and objectively important needs. The range of opportunity implies preferences in choices of life plans (and so does the idea of living a life from the 'inside').[25] Thus it may be very difficult to spell out the "reasonable" in reasonable plans of life. And second, if a reasonable plan cannot be spelled out, then how are we supposed to decide on the kinds of health care included in a package of benefits?

A reasonable plan of life on a straightforward Rawlsian account of justice seems to be any plan of life that does not conflict with the principles of justice he sets out. However, the Rawlsian account does not take into consideration the effect of disease and disability on life plans, while Daniels's account does. On Daniels's account, reasonable life plans just seem to be those to which one is suited given natural attributes and reasonable desires. But this explanation seems to be just begging the question because we have yet to say what "reasonable" means. What is puzzling here is that the exotic dancer's life plan (in terms of a career) could actually be furthered by breast enhancement, but the mastectomy patient's reconstructive surgery can meet only social goals which seem outside the scope of distributive justice. More precisely, it meets a social goal which Daniels explicitly rejects: "The biomedical model thus allows us to draw a fairly sharp line between uses of health-care services to prevent and treat diseases and uses which meet other social goals. The importance of such other goals may be different and may rest on other bases ..."[26] I take it that being more sexually attractive is a goal which lies outside the scope of justice in the distribution of opportunity. Daniels has attempted to draw a line between needs and preferences by first appealing to Rawls's theory, and then modifying the fair equality of opportunity principle to take into account our actual practices.[27] But my analysis of this case shows that specifying "reasonableness" in abstraction from actual cases renders the distinction all but impossible. On the one hand, Daniels wants to insure constraints on public health-care expenditures by appealing to normal species functioning and its effect on the opportunity range. But by broadening his principle he has allowed reasons for services that he actually means to reject. In both the mastectomy case and the enhancement case, the reasons for surgery are sexual attractiveness. The only objective difference between the two cases is that enhancement surgery would actually broaden the woman's opportunity range in respect to careers, but the reconstructive case fails to do even that.

What does this mean? It suggests that on Daniels's account, we may have two choices: either reject the idea of "reasonable" plans, or set out more explicitly what constitutes reasonable plans of life. Rejecting the idea of reasonable plans seems to amount to rejecting any constraints on how limited resources are spent, a consequence that is clearly an unacceptable one.

Daniels's theory, then, must be more explicit about reasonable life plans. Public policy must include some criteria according to which "reasonable" plans are defined. But doing this defeats a central goal of liberal egalitarianism—providing a just framework within which people are free to choose their *own* life plans. This conundrum, itself, is difficult. But it has further implications for the kinds and amounts of health care we might suppose constitute a social obligation. If we do not spell out what plans are reasonable, then we have no way to determine the kinds and amounts of health care goods to which people might be entitled. So, even if the justification for the macroallocation of health care seems plausible, much indeterminacy remains for the application of the justification, i.e., how are we to decide on the microallocation of health care goods?

One answer to this question is to give priority to those whose range of opportunity is most impaired by disease or disability, i.e., the worst off with respect to health. However, given limited resources, we may end up sacrificing even a decent minimum of health care for all in order to pay the fare on the most disadvantaged. The tradeoff seems both unfair and cost ineffective, especially if one considers the tremendous benefits of preventive treatments such as vaccinations for well children and adults.

We might then, consider "worst off" in terms of income and wealth, i.e., those who are on the lowest rung of the index of well-being. But then, of course, the right to health care will not be equal in terms of a national health care plan that pertains to all citizens. Nor are we any closer to knowing what kinds or amounts of health care should be provided to the financially worst off. Presumably we would not want to provide a package so luxurious that the better off are taxed so highly that they can no longer afford to purchase their own private plans (i.e., that their taxes put them on the lowest rung, as well—for that would make health care the insatiable good that would bankrupt even the wealthiest state). But we would want to provide enough to get people back on their feet and enjoying to the extent possible, their lives. How much and what kind, though, remains indeterminate.

A further ramification of indeterminacy arises when we consider that both education and health care are to be governed by the broadened fair equality of opportunity principle. One of the most effective ways to promote equal opportunity, especially for the disadvantaged, is funding various forms of education. Educational funding takes up approximately 6.2 percent of the federal budget,[28] as compared to 6 percent of federal outlays for Medicaid.[29] And if we take seriously the idea of equal opportunity, much more ought to be spent on education. Then we have a serious balancing act between health-care expenditures and educational expenditures. So, again, public policy requires some set guidelines in order to make budgets and plan ahead. But if we do not know what constitutes reasonable plans, and thus do not know what kinds of health care goods might be requirements of a just theory of health care, then we will not know how to divide up the funding for goods governed by the same principle.

To take one last example, Daniels assumes that underlying all mental illnesses interfering with social cooperation or success are physiological causes. But it is certainly unclear to me that all dysfunctional behavior is a product of one's physiology. I think we would have to make some distinctions, as psychiatrists do, that some dysfunctional behavior is more a product of environment, or habit, than a product of faulty genes. Clearly, schizophrenia and bipolar affective disorders have physiological bases. But just as clearly, some violent or dysfunctional behaviors are learned habits. Just as clearly, some dysfunctions are a combination of physiology and habit. And, for all we know, some people might just be evil. On Daniels's theory, would we be required to disentangle these elements and treat only the ones with a physiological basis? And further, if we decided to treat, for want of a better term, "character defects," for how long is society obligated when some refuse to cooperate with their treatment? Referring back again to 'normal species functioning,' it would seem society is obligated to treat so long as the patient resists (or for so long as the patient is not realizing some share of her opportunity range). But then we may just be 'throwing good money after bad,' resulting in providing a less than decent minimum for all. So, it seems that appealing to a normal opportunity range and a biological definition of disease are going to be insufficient in determining actual guidelines for application of the general moral justification because we are unable to make the fine distinctions we had hoped for by appealing to them.

Daniels, himself, is not unaware of this problem. In *Justice and Justification*,[30] he discusses the problem of applying theory to practical ethics. He had thought that his 'modest' revision of the fair equality of opportunity principle would serve as a guideline in the actual determination of health-care benefits provided by institutions. More specifically, he thought that focusing on maintaining normal species functioning would "support a distinction between treatment and enhancement."[31] But it does not do this, at least not in any obvious way. How are we to know, then, what kinds of treatment are required in justice? More specifically, there does not seem to be a principled way of determining the kinds and amounts of health care obliging society under conditions of scare resources.

Daniels now believes that there is not. To quote, "These 'unsolved' rationing problems show just how indeterminate the equal opportunity principle is. It fails to guide our action at a crucial point, where we must design institutions and policies to embody general principles under resource constraints."[32] His belief now is that we must develop fair procedures for making choices in health care design, although little attention has been paid in the literature as to what counts as a fair procedure. One thing seems clear to him now: "We must revise considerably our view about the nature of general distributive principles: they cannot guide action as we might have hoped."[33]

We are thus left not only with principles that are indeterminate in guiding actions, but indeterminacy concerning the most productive way to proceed in deciding public policy. In the next chapter, I address Michael Walzer's proposal that the proper procedure, or method, for determining public policy is by examining our historical and present practices in order to tease out their meanings for the people who actually decide upon and live with their choices. His proposal, too, may be interpreted as broadly based on the idea of equal opportunity. But as a communitarian, Walzer is more concerned with health care and its relation to securing equal citizenship status. His claim is that citizens have shown through their practices and traditions that certain goods are needs, one of which is health care. Once a good has been established as a need, claims Walzer, to be left out of the distribution of such a good is tantamount to being a second-class citizen. He thus distinguishes himself from the liberal egalitarian in the sense that his claim does not rest on the pursuit of individual life plans, but rather on the opportunity of citizens to equally realize the good of citizenship in the community of which they are a part.

CHAPTER 4

MICHAEL WALZER: THE COMMUNITARIAN

We ended the last chapter with the dismaying conclusion that general distributive principles are of little help in guiding our actions under concrete circumstances. One might speculate upon several reasons for this result. First, the principle of fair equality of opportunity under which Daniels has subsumed health-care provision may simply be the wrong one, or his broadened version of it might have rendered the principle too susceptible to confusions and indeterminacy. Second, we might believe that any general principle is simply too general for the specific and concrete decisions that need to be made in our complex, everyday lives. As such, general principles can serve, at best, as only vague frameworks or criterion for the design of institutions. But they were never meant to provide concrete guidelines in the first place. A third possibility is that general principles explain and systematize what are thought to be universal values and moral intuitions fairly well, but once we attempt to apply them to a particular society we find that they may lack coherence with the actual practices decided upon by the citizens of that community. The last of these possibilities differs from the second in that the last is actually meant to provide concrete guidelines, but fails to do so in a fashion coherent with the historical and cultural practices of a particular community, while the second simply turns out to be too vague for practical use even though it resonates with the values of the community.

There remains a fourth possibility. This position maintains that the meanings of social goods generate principles that may or may not be universal, but that the principles possess legitimacy only when they express the internal logic of the meanings of goods relative to a particular society. That is, the legitimacy of principles relies on the deep and inclusive meanings of goods and practices. Thus, on this proposal, social goods with their thick and socially textured meanings are prior to the principles which they generate.

It is the last possibility with which Michael Walzer is concerned in *Spheres of Justice—A Defense of Pluralism and Equality*.[1] The argument in this book presents one communitarian view of distributive justice. It is centrally concerned with the idea that the different goods conceived and created in a society possess different social meanings, and because they do, they ought to be distributed according to the principles their meanings generate. Since the meanings of these goods generate different principles, it follows for Walzer, that no one principle nor any one set of principles can act as sufficient guidelines for the just distribution of goods. Walzer especially rejects the liberal individualist method of adopting value-laden, universalistic principles in abstraction from particular communities.[2] It is his contention that even if universal principles are discoverable, they will not reflect the rich, lived-in character of the values that have evolved in a single society and which constitute the form of life for the company of people in that society. Rather than attempting to discover universal principles, Walzer believes that the principles guiding distributions of goods ought to be radically particularistic to the history and culture of a community. As such, Walzer's work both represents a rejection of the methodology employed by Rawls, Daniels and Green and argues for a plurality of distributive principles appropriate to the various spheres of goods conceived, created and distributed by a particular community.

Walzer argues that the premises with which individualism begins fail to capture the nature of individuals situated as they are in a particular community. The individualist, most notably Kant and neo-Kantians, typically starts with the image of individuals as free and equal, able to choose their goals in life largely uninfluenced by the values of their community. It is precisely this ability to choose life goals unencumbered by the values, practices and traditions of this or that community that is highly prized by the individualist. The communitarian, on the other hand, says separating the individual from her goals is precisely the wrong way to understand persons, for they are constituted by the community of which they are a part and are not free to choose their aims unencumbered by their social background. The values of the community determine in a large way, the goals at which individuals aim. Thus, the individual and her goals cannot be so easily separated as the individualist believes, nor should they be. To attempt to do so has the effect of separating the individual from the values she holds as a member of a particular community. This 'unencumbered' conception of the person, argues the communitarian, fails to make sense of both human behavior and social life as we know it.[3]

For his part, Walzer argues that when we conceive social goods as merely means to individual ends, we fail to take into account the meanings they already possess for individuals of a particular community. Goods are not simply instrumental to some life goal, possessing no value of their own. Rather, social goods are imbued with meanings and values particular to a community. Our social world is made up of the things that we have first conceived and created. And because goods are a social creation, they already possess a shared meaning. Thus rather than starting out, as Rawls has done, with an abstract conception of the individual from which a 'thin' theory of primary social goods follows, Walzer's starting point is from a 'thick' theory of social goods.

Walzer's central argument for his method of arriving at a just distribution of social goods starts with the premise that people are culture-producing—they conceive and create social goods with a specific purpose in mind. Each and every social good thus possesses a shared meaning in a particular society and its distribution is implied by its shared understanding. Because goods are created in the context of a society with a specific purpose in mind, they are valued by the *community* in contrast to the individual. That is, goods have value for the individual just because of the wider value and meaning they have for the community. And, in fact, Walzer claims that people are so intrinsically constituted by their possessions that their concrete identities are formed "because of the way they conceive and create, and then possess and employ social goods."[4] For instance, Walzer's understanding of the importance of religion in the Middle Ages is that the "curing of souls" was a socially recognized common need; as such, it was publicly provided so that every Christian "had an equal chance at salvation, catechism for the young, compulsory communion, and so on."[5]
Since different goods have been conceived and created for different purposes, they possess different social meanings. These meanings, themselves, determine their distribution. "Distributive criteria and

arrangements are intrinsic not to the good-in-itself but to the social good. If we understand what it is, what it means to those for whom it is a good, we understand how, by whom, and for what reasons it ought to be distributed."[6] Thus, distributions of goods are just or unjust relative to their social meaning. Those meanings are historical and contextual in nature, i.e., their distinct meanings have evolved over time and they are embedded in a particular community. When meanings of goods are distinct, it follows for Walzer that their distributions must be autonomous. These autonomous distributions thus constitute spheres of distribution. Walzer argues, then, for a plurality of distributive spheres, each constituted by the meanings of different social goods and each governed by a principle generated by the internal logic of the meanings of goods. According to Walzer, when goods are distributed by meanings other than their deeply and widely shared social understandings, unjust distributions arise.

Walzer contends that when goods are distributed by meanings other than their shared social meanings, it is often the result of dominance by a prized social good held in monopoly against others. The idea is this: he claims that buried in our social meanings already lies the idea of justice and equality. While liberal theories try to work out an egalitarian society by attempting to level the differences between individuals by distributing dominant social goods more evenly, Walzer claims that what is needed is not to reduce the monopoly of certain goods held by individuals. Rather, what is needed is to first distribute goods by their meanings, and second, to make sure that dominant goods—say money—do not operate outside their appropriate sphere. Money is an appropriate medium of exchange in free markets, but it is inappropriate in other spheres, according to Walzer. When a dominant good such as money brings with it the distribution of goods outside the boundary of the free market, individuals gain a monopoly not just in the free market, but in spheres external to the free market. It is not *per se* monopolistic holdings within a given sphere to which Walzer objects. Rather, it is the conversion of a dominant good from one sphere to another that makes for unjust distributions. One such example comes to mind: the good of credit cards. Credit cards were first conceived and created for the purpose of purchasing certain goods, typically luxury items, or 'long-distance' items such as airline tickets or catalogue merchandise. Over time, the meaning of credit cards has expanded such that they have become means of identification and a symbol of material success and independence. Moreover, the stakes keep getting higher—possessing *just* a credit card is no longer symbolic of success—rather, possessing a 'gold' or better, a 'platinum' card is necessary. And those without a credit card are in an important sense, denied a great many of the benefits of the community. One may not, for instance, rent a car without a major credit card in hand. Thus, possessing credit cards in the US works as identification in the economic community (it is hard to do business without one) or they identify one as among the successful, or both. In short, the possession of credit cards in the US has come to constitute in some measure our identities. But for Walzer, I believe that he would say that since the possession of credit cards has crossed the boundary of the free market, that the use of them has been corrupted. Thus, when individuals have monopolistic control of a dominant good and that good converts into goods from other spheres of distribution, then we have a tyrannical form of distribution in which "the rich grind the faces of the poor, impose their poverty upon them, command their deferential behavior."[7] For Walzer then, egalitarian communities are distinguished by freedom from tyranny exercised by some members because of their possession and then inappropriate use of a dominant good. In other words, when the boundaries between different distributive spheres are breached, we have a situation in which the standing of poor members of the community is marginalized and they fail to reap the full benefits of membership.

Failure to realize full-membership benefits in a community, itself, violates the meaning of what Walzer understands to be an implicit social contract. His interpretation of the social contract is that people have come together for the sake of survival and well-being which require a common effort. They are thus already committed to 'dividing, exchanging and sharing' among themselves the social goods that make this possible. In view of this commitment, people have strong duties to provide needed goods to one another, for they have cut themselves off from others and are committed to sharing a common way of life. The social contract "is an agreement to redistribute the resources of the members in accordance with some shared understanding of their needs, subject to ongoing political determination in detail."[8] First among these commitments is mutual provision of security and welfare. His reading of the social contract thus involves a claim that there exists a special relation among members of a community that requires providing for the needs of members when they are unable to provide for themselves. At the same time, mutual provision promotes the value of community. The social contract is thus a two-way street: communal provision teaches people the value of membership in a community, and at the same time, 'love of country' arises out of mutual provision.

Since for Walzer, needs acquire a particular meaning within any historically and culturally conditioned city or community, the shape of the distribution of security and welfare will vary. Walzer's vision of the social contract, then, entails that communal provision of needed goods is in accordance with shared understandings. To be sure, some goods are needed absolutely, but their priorities *vis* à *vis* each other and how much of them we owe to one another cannot be known ahead of time, and independently of the customs, traditions, and actual political determinations of citizens. We might think, for instance, that the meaning of food is 'reiterated' across all lines of time and space. Yet, even such staples as bread possess different meanings depending on the culture. "Bread is the staff of life, the body of Christ, the symbol of the Sabbath, the means of hospitality, and so on."[9] Thus, for Walzer, there can be no single principle of distribution decided upon in abstraction from a particular society that is, at the same time, true to its thick cultural meaning.

This vision of the distribution of basic goods obviously is at variance with a Rawlsian conception of social goods that is determined in abstraction from the actual practices of particular communities. Rather than deriving principles from a context of deeply embedded, enmeshed and widespread understandings of social goods and of what the good life consists in, Rawls attempts to derive principles from a 'thin' theory of goods. That is, a Rawlsian conception of justice argues for a distribution of goods impartial to particular conceptions of the good, but which at the same time expresses fundamental values, such as freedom and equality, that are reiterated across most democratic, pluralistic societies. Hence, a Rawlsian conception of justice explicitly rejects distributing goods by the decisions that citizens have already made, it rejects a distribution of goods that would favor any one conception of the good, and it rejects the idea of particularity in respect to values. Rather, so long as a state is democratic and pluralistic in nature, then Rawls's theory should apply whether that state is the US, or any other democratic, pluralistic state. However, Walzer insists that it is hard to argue that the actual decisions made by citizens in a particular state to spend public funds on goods in accordance with their thick understandings is mistaken.

This interpretation of the social contract as a mutual agreement to provide needed goods to one another leads Walzer to examine what goods a given community such as the US might consider needs of citizens. His understanding of the agreement thus suggests to him that the appropriate principle governing mutual provision is the principle of need. Needs, according to Walzer are *socially* recognized goods thought necessary to the common life of a community. Or as Walzer puts it, "all that is required to make [a good] morally necessary is the development of a "want" so widely and deeply felt that it can plausibly be said that it is the want not of this or that person alone but of the community generally."[10] As such, it would violate the meanings of the goods constituting the sphere of welfare and security should they be distributed according to merit or free-market principles. The idea here is that the social and moral logic of some goods makes them needs. If we pay attention to the purpose of, for instance, giving food, we find that we 'give it to needy persons to relieve hunger.' On the other hand, if we hand out promotions, we find that those are distributed on the basis of merit. To further the comparison, the inner logic of luxury boats puts them in a distributive sphere governed by free market principles. However, needy persons do not have to 'stage a performance nor pass an exam' to obtain food—all that is required is that they need it. And, Walzer contends, "once the community undertakes to provide some needed good, it must provide it to all the members who need it in proportion to their needs."[11] By this Walzer means that the only acceptable limitations on provision of needs are available resources, and not money or desert because those are the wrong exchange mediums. Walzer does not insist, of course, that there are absolutely unanimous decisions about social goods that fall under the province of communal provisions. He admits that disagreements will arise about both the particular goods to be provided and the extent of the provision. But once the members of a community understand that such-and-such a good is needed by members in order to sustain their membership in the community, the sphere of welfare and security must include it. Failure to do so will violate both the understanding of community as mutual provision and the understanding of the needed good in question.

Health Care in the United States

According to Walzer, one such failing is the lack of provision of health care to all needy members of the US community. He argues that the meaning of health care in the US has evolved to that of a needed good, but that its communal provision does not measure up to the internal requirements of the sphere of welfare and security—that it must be provided equally to all members of the US. The argument for this conclusion traces the shift in attitudes and historical practices of medicine. Modern medical technology made advances only after the Second World War. Prior to that time, health care was more a luxury item than a needed item. As a luxury item affordable to mostly the wealthy, it was appropriate for it to be distributed according to the free market. However, Walzer admits that its meaning, even then, was more complex. He finds evidence suggesting that physicians had a bad conscience with respect to serving only the wealthy, and it's his understanding that this bad conscience was because of medicine's inner logic: that it should be distributed in proportion to illness, and not to wealth. Because of this bad conscience, some physicians have always contributed some free care to the poor, as well as feeling obligated to help victims in an emergency irrespective of their financial status or, I suppose, whether they can give proof of health insurance. Nonetheless, the provision of health care has been delivered from the Middle Ages until recently, mainly on a free market basis and understood as a luxury, basically because medicine had not been all that successful in dealing with illness and disability. Indeed, people placed little faith in the ability of medicine to cure illness. Hence, there was little political demand by citizens to replace the distribution of health care by the free market with communal provision.

However, according to Walzer, there has been a reversal of meaning in respect to health care, from the free market to communal provision. His explanation for this reversal is that there has been a major shift in common understandings of the salvation of souls and bodies. The West has lost faith in the ability of religion to save our souls for eternal life, but has gradually gained faith in modern medical technology to save our bodies. In earlier times, there was a socially recognized need for eternity and social efforts were made to see that salvation was 'widely and equally distributed.' There were churches in every neighborhood, or in their absence, I might add, there were circuit preachers making the word of God available to all.

Walzer interprets modern practices to indicate a shift in attitudes. We no longer make religion as available to citizens as we used to, according to him. Because of advances in medical technology, longevity has become a socially recognized need. Churches have been replaced by physicians, hospitals and clinics in every neighborhood in a greater effort to see that medicine is widely and equally distributed and that every citizen has an equal chance at a long and healthy life. We not only focus on the curing of bodies, we also focus on prevention of disease through regular check-ups and public health measures. Our public education institutions insist on compulsory vaccinations for school children and personnel. There is, in short, a greater faith in medicine to cure our bodies than in religion to cure our souls. According to Walzer, illness and disease have "come to be seen as a plague, and since the plague can be dealt with, it *must* be dealt with."[12] But because fighting disease is expensive, it requires a common commitment.

This shift in attitudes has its parallel in a shift in institutions. We now license physicians in a state-sponsored attempt to regulate the quality of medical care. In addition, the state invests huge sums of money in medical schools and voluntary hospitals. To Walzer, these practices represent a recognition that medicine is no longer a private pursuit. More evidence supporting Walzer's interpretation of health care as a need lies in state-subsidized research, training for physicians, providing equipment for hospitals, regulating insurance schemes, and the Medicare and Medicaid programs. To Walzer, these measures represent "'the contrivance of human wisdom to provide for human wants.' And all that is required to make it morally necessary is the development of a 'want' so widely and deeply felt that it can plausibly be said that it is the want not of this or that person alone but of the community generally."[13] Thus, according to Walzer's readings of communal provision and the shift in attitudes and practices of health care in the US, health care must be provided equally to all the members of the community 'in ways that respect their membership,' i.e., in ways that do not exclude them from a communally recognized need. For otherwise members, "are locked into an inferior position."[14]

Clearly Walzer's reading of the meaning of health care is not reflected in our actual practices. But the principle of need acts not only as a standard for communal provision, it also acts as a principle of criticism. Walzer thus criticizes our actual practices. He notes that while we have Medicare, Medicaid and other forms of communal provision which are intended to provide at least minimally decent health care, there are still people who are either left out of the distribution, or whose provision is below minimal standards. And this circumstance, insists Walzer, is inconsistent with the decisions we have already made with respect to health care. So long as federal, state and local governments fund medical research, "build hospitals, and pay the fees of doctors in private practice, the services that these expenditures underwrite must be equally available to all citizens."[15] In other words, since federal, state and local governments have already committed communal funds to health care just because it is understood as part of the sphere of communal provision, then an unequal distribution of it (with the middle class and the wealthy receiving more and better health care) is unjust because it violates its social understanding. Thus, Walzer insists that the less advantaged must have the same access to health care and physicians as the more advantaged.

Further, he points out that so long as free enterprise operates in medical care wealth will continue to dominate in this part of the sphere of security and welfare, and that circumstance is in violation of its social meaning because individuals will be cared for in proportion to their ability to pay rather than their illness. If health care were a luxury, then unequal distributions would not matter, but according to Walzer's understanding, health care is a socially recognized need. As such, it matters a great deal when some citizens are left out of the distribution because physicians and hospitals have "become such massively important features of contemporary life that to be cut off from the help they provide is not only dangerous but also degrading."[16] When the meaning of a good has come to represent in an important way part of what it means to be a citizen of a society, not sharing in that good is tantamount to being in the position of a shirt-tail relative whom the rest of the family disavows. One is not quite out of the community, but by no means is one a fully valued member either.

To summarize, Walzer argues for a plurality of distributive principles, each of which is to be generated by the meaning a social good has in a particular society, and each of which is appropriate to a distinct sphere of social goods. Distributive justice obtains when the boundaries between the spheres remain fixed by their meanings. A citizen may rightly possess more of one sort of good so long as that good does not bring with it a good from another sphere only because of the possession of the first good. But when the possession of, say, money brings with it a greater provision of socially recognized needs such as health care, then Walzer will say that boundaries between different spheres have been unjustly breached. It is then that citizens have a right to complain about the justice of distributions, for they no longer match their common understandings. But just the bare fact that there may be a wide gap with respect to income and wealth does not justify complaints. It is not the overall situations of citizens to which Walzer draws our attention, but rather their situations *vis* à *vis* the common meanings of goods. With respect to health care, Walzer claims its meaning as a need puts it squarely in the sphere of security and welfare. Thus, even if citizens do not have the financial means to purchase private insurance, according to Walzer they should still have access to the important good of health care, in accordance to what he understands its common meaning to be.

Whose Interpretations?

Walzer admits that his interpretation of the meaning of health care is controversial. Most notably, in his discussion of health care as a commodity distributed by physicians as free-enterprise agents, he admits to controversy around the edges. He insists, however, that the practices and attitudes of US citizens provide evidence for his interpretation of the meaning of health care as a need.

No one, of course, denies that health care is a need. Walzer is probably correct that when citizens are left out of the distribution of health care it jeopardizes not only their health but their standing in the community. There are two important questions one can ask, though, concerning Walzer's interpretation. These questions concern, in turn, the various meanings and purposes of health care in the US, and the meanings of justice, itself, in a pluralistic society.

To begin, most of us would admit that health care has other meanings and purposes as well, i.e., the premise with which Walzer starts—that people conceive and create social goods with *only one* specific purpose in mind—seems to be false. First to come to mind in respect to meanings and purposes is Daniels's claim that health care protects the range of opportunities and individually chosen goals of citizens. Of course, this purpose of health care might roughly be defined as a need. But it depends on how one defines "need." It might be defined as necessary to one's life and health, but it might also be defined as a means to some other goal, such as improving one's prospects for a job or improving one's appearance, and so on. So it seems to me that simply saying something is a 'need' fails to make the finer-grained distinctions that we, in fact, make. Under this latter interpretation of health care, I want to stipulate that while need plays a role in communal provision, the more distinctive meaning of it at this level is that it serves as a means to jobs, education and training which in turn allow an individual latitude in pursuing a life style she finds fulfilling. An example might prove useful here. A medical condition such as defective vision is normally not life-threatening; an individual may very well go through life using eye glasses. But this same individual may still not be able to pursue her self-chosen goal without corrective surgery. Airline pilots come to mind in this regard. In the past, the Federal Aviation Agency ruled out pilots for commercial purposes whose vision was worse than 20/200 without correction. However, the FAA now approves those pilots who have had their vision corrected by laser (and other) surgeries. Clearly, these individuals need surgery to pursue their goals, but we would hardly say they need surgery for life or health reasons. Thus, Walzer's concept of need is overly-broad because it fails to distinguish between different meanings of need. Clearly, failure to distinguish between different conceptions of need will result in distributive schemes untrue to the more subtly nuanced decisions that the US has already made. The example of laser surgery makes this point: someone may say she *needs* surgery so that she can qualify for pilot training, yet to my knowledge that sort of health care is not publicly funded. So, it seems reasonable to infer that the US stops short of providing just any health care proclaimed to be a need. Walzer may very well say that is exactly what he means: that laser surgery is not a need because it has yet to be a "want" deeply and widely felt. But I do not believe that just saying something is a need because it is deeply and widely wanted will make his case. Rather, we require an explanation of what the need is for—what purpose does it serve? In the case of laser surgery, the purpose seems to be fulfilling a specific individual goal. The same may be said about various cosmetic surgeries. Yet other treatments, such as cataract surgery, are needed because they promote a more basic, general purpose; namely: that of an equal opportunity to pursue not just this or that specific goal, but opportunity in general. Thus, the notion of "need" *simpliciter* will not carry the argument. The question is not, then, Is a treatment a need? but rather, What is the treatment a need for? What purpose does it serve?

Equally obvious is the fact that health care offers a way to continue life even after life ceases to provide opportunities as we normally think of them: for instance, people in a persistent vegetative state on life support systems can hardly be considered in the competition for jobs. Health care also has the ability to either cosmetically restore or enhance physical characteristics. We might also plausibly believe that another purpose of medical care is to either increase productivity of workers for the common good, or to reward them for their contribution to the country's economy. We might even understand some health care as a symbol of our freedom to choose the ways in which we wish to spend our money. These few examples indicate the problems we encounter on Walzer's theory, for the social meaning of health care is not quite so singular as Walzer claims it to be.

Perhaps the reason Walzer believes that health care has only one meaning rests on a hidden assumption: he seems to assume that spheres of distribution with their internal principles lie above and beyond our actual practices—somewhat on the order of Plato's ideal forms.[17] In his discussion of security and welfare, he says that the 'social contract is an agreement to reach decisions together about what goods are necessary to our common life.'[18] It is not the case that Walzer assumes there are a given set of goods necessary to a common life, but rather that there *are* goods, whatever they may be, required for a common life. He likewise assumes there is a sphere of money in which commodities "beyond what is communally provided,"[19] are properly bought and sold. Further, he says that even though the commodities, themselves, change according to a culture the "market is standard,"[20] i.e., the market has always existed. These assumptions of Walzer seem to be fair enough; for we do, indeed, see divisions between the ways different goods are distributed. But what seems to be an unsafe assumption is that there is no interaction between these spheres that does not, at the same time, violate their boundaries. Thus, based on the assumption that boundaries between spheres should be inviolable, Walzer seems compelled to interpret the meaning of a good in a singular way, placing one good in one sphere and another in some other sphere. Thus, each social good we conceive and create is assigned to one and only one sphere—admissions to medical schools and positions of authority are assigned to the sphere of office, with talent or qualification as its internal principle. Commodities are assigned to the market sphere, and so on.

I want to suggest that Walzer's assumption has led him to limit the illustrations with which he supports his interpretation of the meaning of health care. If one assumes there exist these bounded spheres into which each and every good neatly fits, then one will tend to look for illustrations to support that view. However, that assumption has the effect of closing off other possible arrangements. One might see, as Daniels has, the interaction between different spheres—the spheres of health care and equal opportunity. Or, as I have seen, the interaction between health care and the market, or the interaction between health care and merit based on employment. But Walzer's view expressly forbids these interactions, for they breach the boundaries of his preconceived spheres. But given my analysis of the distribution of health care, it seems much more plausible that the meaning of health care is complex, fitting into several different spheres rather than a single one. Thus, despite his evidence for health care as a need to which all members should have equal access, there is greater evidence contradicting the idea that health care's only meaning is that of a need. We come nowhere close to distributing breast implants on the level of communal provision, nor do we communally provide expensive diagnostic procedures such as magnetic resonance imaging, and so on. But Walzer ignores or dismisses this other evidence which suggests competing, and equally valid interpretations of the meanings of health care.

One cannot easily dismiss, however, some of Walzer's examples supporting his view. For instance, it is true that the Medicare and Medicaid programs are federally funded government programs. It is equally true that medical research, hospitals, and training physicians are subsidized by government funds. These practices might suggest that we, as US citizens, have decided that health care should be delivered equally to everyone on the basis of need. And when one considers that even the care of the wealthy relies on research to which we have all contributed, it might plausibly be thought that health care has become a 'want so widely and deeply felt' that it is a need which ought to be communally provided equally to everyone.

Yet there remains the possibility that we have decided that the disadvantaged are entitled to just the amount of health care that they receive under Medicaid, and that the elderly must subsidize their Medicare benefits if they wish more health care, and that the employed are entitled to more health care because of their contribution to society, and that the wealthy are entitled to even more just because they either contribute more to the general fund through their taxes, or because out-of-pocket payments express the ability to dispose of one's income in ways one sees fit, or both.[21]

And to paraphrase Walzer, it is hard to argue that the decision to distribute health care on these alternative bases is wrong, for they constitute fully one half of the distribution of health care in the US. His selection of examples thus seems unduly biased by his own perspective, and not necessarily reflective of the totality of actual distributive practices.

Given these alternative bases of health-care delivery, a more plausible interpretation of health care's meaning is that it is mixed. The principle of equal opportunity seems to be the basis of distribution with respect to Medicare, Medicaid and the various state and local agencies. Purchasing health care, or health care insurance, above and beyond employer-based provision represents the free enterprise system, and employer-based insurance may plausibly fall under the rubric of merit. Obviously, within each of these categories one could claim 'need' depending on one's perspective and preferences. The very wealthy might claim need for health insurance that covers the costs of cryogenic treatment. And one would hardly need to convince any employee that besides health insurance as a benefit, it is also a needed good. There are thus a great variety of interpretations of health care as a need, and it is not clear to me that the use of the term "need" makes the finer-grained distinctions between our actual three-pronged distributive scheme. But that the actual distribution is roughly divided under three distributive principles may well reflect our recognition of the values represented by them. Or, in other words, it may well reflect our belief that since health care is so diverse, this is the nearest we can come to justice in the distribution of health care.

At any rate, it is hard to argue that our actual distribution of health care is not provided by different mechanisms in accordance to its different meanings. Thus, the distribution of health care may very well spill over from one sphere to another without violating its meaning in the US; and the moral necessity of all of it being communally provided does not automatically follow as Walzer believes. Of course, the moral necessity of a three-pronged distribution of health care does not automatically follow from the actual distribution either. In the next chapter I shall advance arguments to the effect that if actual health-care delivery met its ideal goals, i.e., if it covered everyone who it is supposed to under each distributive principle, then our system of delivery would be a just distribution. In order to do this, I shall have to give arguments not only about our actual practices in respect to health care, but I shall have to say something about the justice of such an enterprise. Clearly the justice of a distribution cannot rely solely on a single interpretation of meaning, for there are many interpretations. And Walzer offers no methodological premises to which we can appeal in order to settle which interpretation is correct, or which distribution is just.

The second important question which Walzer's interpretation raises concerns justice, itself. Walzer seems to misunderstand the real issue. It is not that we debate the meaning of health care, for we all have a rough idea about its meaning.[22] It is rather that we debate what justice, itself, requires as to the degree and extent of the whole complex of the distributive scheme of health care. Broadening or narrowing the context in which we consider justice, will yield different distributive decisions.[23] A very narrow context may yield either Walzer's position—that health care ought to be distributed equally to everyone—or it may yield a libertarian position—that all health care should be distributed as a commodity. A wider context that considers the multitude of meanings which health care possesses may very well yield the result that justice requires a much more complex distribution than either Walzer or a strict libertarian cares to admit. Given the diversity of meanings of both health care and justice, it seems to me that we are more true to our historically and culturally situated society when we broaden the context in which we consider both health-care practices and the various meanings of justice. We are a pluralistic nation, and because of that, the concept of justice, itself, possesses various meanings. Ask the students in any one classroom what "justice" means, and one is likely to get a variety of answers—some tending strongly to a libertarian view, and some leaning far more in the direction of redistributive schemes which favor a rigid equality, and still others who believe that market principles ought to be tempered by the value of compassion. It thus seems that the wisest course would be to broaden the context in which we consider the justice of distributions, thereby not closing off the possibility of making compromises between competing interpretations of the meaning of distributive justice, nor foreclosing on the interrelations between health care and other social goods.[24] It just might be the case that our existing distribution of health care reflects both the various meanings of distributive justice and the compromises which living in a pluralistic society entails.

One reason Walzer may have foreclosed on the wide meanings of health care is that he seems to assume a more, rather than less, homogeneous population that for the most part agrees upon actual distributions. We might think, then, that his methodology would get us closer to a package of health care needs for US citizens (the kind and amount) than Daniels's proposal. However, that is not Walzer's position. He rather maintains that those decisions are "subject to ongoing political determination in detail."[25] In other places, Walzer states that if communities are so divided that their "sensibilities and intuitions aren't readily shared, (then) the sharing takes place in smaller units...we should look for some way to adjust distributive decisions to the requirements of those units."[26] Here, if the understanding of health care varies from region to region in the US, then different regions may distribute health care differently, subject to political adjustments for these differences at the federal level. But that result is hardly consistent with Walzer's view of a national health care plan. I want to suggest that it is not regional differences that divide citizens about the distribution of health care, for we are a highly mobile nation which uses television as a platform for debate about national decisions, in effect making the boundaries between geographical regions much less rigid. But rather, we dispute as a nation about the meaning of justice because of our cultural plurality. Thus, we need not be driven to the extreme of dividing into smaller distributional units in order to be just or true to our social meanings, but rather need to find a way to compromise and adjust meanings such that one view does not dominate over equally valid interpretations.

Walzer's train of thinking seems to be this: he assumes more, rather than less, homogeneity about the social meaning of health care. From the assumption that all, or at least most, health care is a need, he seems to assume a minimal amount of dissent about the kind and amount of health care (he says it should be provided in proportion to need, not merit and so on, and that its only constraint should be actual resources). Now, it is probably true that we all know roughly what health care means, but it is precisely this roughness that is the problem. There is such a broad range of health-care treatments that it cannot plausibly be the case that health care possesses a unique and decisive meaning. We thus need to make more finely grained distinctions between the various meanings and purposes of health care. Not all health-care treatments are needs; some are clearly preferences for which the US community presumably does not believe it is responsible.

Of course, Walzer may very well say that his main point is that health care is a need, and once that's been understood, we can leave the package of benefits (how much and what kind of health care) open to democratic debate. So, he may continue, there is really very little difference between his principle of need and the principle of equal opportunity that I propose. Otherwise put, both principles are open to democratic debate as to amounts and kinds of health care. But I want to point out that it does make a difference. The principle of equal opportunity at least narrows the range of the debate. It is not hard to imagine the wrangling when the notion of "need" drives the debate. And in the end, I believe that we would be forced to ask, not just if a certain type of health care is a need, but what is it needed for? And, I believe that finally, in addition to treatments that save lives or prevent public health threats, we would include treatments the purpose of which are to promote an equal opportunity for jobs and careers in general.[27]

But it is not just that health care has various meanings; it is also the case that we live in a pluralistic nation in which some individuals place a greater emphasis on some meaning of justice and other individuals place a greater emphasis on another meaning of justice. These different emphases result in different ideas about what justice requires in the way of distributions. Thus, if we mean to be true to the multiple meanings of health care and the different emphases placed on meanings of justice, we need to take into account a much broader context for understanding than Walzer does. My main point here is that because of the plurality of meanings with respect to both health care and justice, US citizens have decided that a three-pronged distribution of health care is the best they can do by way of a fair distribution. In other words, at some level we acknowledge that when we must make decisions in real time about public policy, we recognize the need to compromise between competing meanings and values.

And perhaps compromise is the deepest and most widely shared meaning which we recognize in respect to the justice of policy decisions. A pluralistic nation respects, because it must if it expects to continue as a nation, the idea that compromise is the essence of settling disputes between competing meanings of values, practices and institutions. It just may be that the deepest meaning of justice is compromise between its competing meanings. That is to say, individuals in pluralistic nations may recognize that they must stand back a little from their own interpretations of justice in order to make the claim that a distribution is just because it respects to some degree their own views, but respects at the same time and to some degree, other views.

Moreover, it seems to me that compromise between competing ideas of justice and meanings of social goods overcomes a problem posed by Walzer's interpretation of health care. He takes our social practices and institutions and then attempts to tease out the meanings of goods relevant to them. But he ignores the fact that US citizens may not consent to these practices to the same degree and for the same reasons. Some comply out of disinterest, some comply because they hold a minority voice, and some comply because it serves their interests. Joshua Cohen[28] makes the point that despite our practices, we may not be equally committed to the values underlying them. Yet, if we take seriously, and make explicit, that justice requires compromise between competing meanings rather than insisting dogmatically that social goods possess one dominant meaning, we are much more likely to remain true to the differences in social meanings that are the mark of cultural plurality. Thus, we need not give up on the idea of social meanings. Rather, justice would be better served if we cast our net more broadly and deeply for the more nuanced and diverse interpretations of meanings in health care and distributive principles.

CHAPTER 5

PRINCIPLES AND PRACTICES

One of the observations made in the last chapter is that the American people have not decided that communal provision of health care is the only appropriate method of distribution. According to a recent study, 58 percent of the population in California relies on employment-based insurance,[1] while older government statistics put the figure at 30 percent nationwide. Whatever the real percent is, it is clear that our actual practices of health care distribution imply more than one principle of distribution. Thus, Walzer's understanding of health care solely as a need does not make the distinctions that we find among the different prongs of health care distribution in the US. Of course, Walzer may believe that the second two prongs are failures to distribute health care by its deep meaning. But I shall argue in this chapter, first, that Walzer's interpretation of health care is biased, and because of that he has selected illustrations of health care practices from too narrow a context. A broader context in which to consider a range of illustrations, I shall argue, is by far more representative of our actual practices and will give a truer picture of the meanings of health care. Second, I shall argue that Walzer's selectivity of examples has led him to accept only one principle of distribution, but in view of a more accurate representation of our actual practices, several principles of distribution are appropriate. And finally, I shall set out a somewhat idealized version of our actual practice of health care distribution according to which health care is provided to everyone as implied by our practices and the principles underlying them.

Practices

Let us begin by taking several health care practices that seem to be clear instances of need. In a broad and undifferentiated sense, we can suppose some treatment is a need if the illness either threatens life, or if the illness poses a public health threat, or if the treatment prevents serious illnesses, or if it holds the possibility of restoring one to a functioning capacity. Both insurance schemes and public funding cover expenses for some potentially life-threatening illnesses. An infected appendix, many forms of cancer, strep throat, kidney disease and pneumonia come to mind because they have the potential to threaten one's life, and in some cases even the flu can threaten life as well as pose a public health crisis. But in addition, illnesses that threaten one's life obviously have the potential to threaten our functioning capacities. It might be thought, then, that neither insurance schemes nor public funding would be denied to cover these treatments, since health care is a need, on this account. There are limitations, however, even with these clear examples. For instance, within certain constraints an insurance scheme might not accept a new subscriber with a history of cancer even though medical treatment might very well be classified as a need, and public funding in this case may well be limited to certain forms of treatment even though an alternative treatment may be far more efficacious. Thus, the notion of need, by itself, does not necessarily entail that a treatment believed to be a need will be provided on that basis.

More controversial forms of treatment needs are exemplified by prolonging the life of a patient diagnosed in a persistent vegetative state. The amount of treatment provided by health insurance schemes is normally limited by common practices such as refusing coverage for a respirator when the patient is elderly and medical consensus has been reached that the condition is irreversible. If the family refuses to give consent to remove the patient from life support, public funds take over. However, public forms of assistance in these cases usually are limited to "comfort care," with more aggressive treatments ruled out because of their expense. Thus, even if family members insist that their loved one 'needs' more aggressive treatment, both public funding agencies and insurance schemes draw a line between what they consider a need and what private individuals consider a need. Still, if private individuals can afford, and are willing, to purchase out of their own funds more aggressive treatments because they see them as a needed good, then normally they will find hospitals that are willing to sell those services.

In the case of public health threats such as the flu or polio, often various clinics offer vaccinations free of charge, but just as frequently there is at least a minimal charge. For instance, campus student health services offer health insurance to their population. Many of their services are covered under their insurance scheme, but students pay an additional fee for flu vaccinations. But in other places such as a working environment, often vaccinations are offered free of charge even without an insurance scheme covering their employees.[2] Still other places of employment include in their employees' insurance package vaccinations for flu, polio, and so on. While these vaccinations seem to qualify as needs (according to the broad definition), they are distributed by principles other than that of need as well: the principles of merit and free exchange also play a role.

Kinds of health care other than those that we might think of as a need in the broad sense, and which *are* covered by insurance schemes might include treatment for certain skin conditions, on-going treatment for addictions, reconstructive mammoplasty and infertility. These examples might be controversial, for in some sense they may be thought of as a need in the sense I have set out. But I think, strictly speaking, they are neither necessary for life, nor as a public health measure, nor do they prevent serious illnesses or affect our capacity to function. Some of these examples might meet other social goals, such as having children, or being more attractive. And at least in respect to treatment of addictions, there are alternatives to medical treatments such as 12-step programs which are at least as, and probably more, successful than medical care in the recovery process.[3]

These examples suggest that many insurance schemes do not limit coverage to treatments that are a need as I have defined it, although those treatments are included. On the other hand, they do not appear to be merely luxury items. I expect that we could say that these treatments contribute to the well-being of people by either providing life-saving or curative treatments, making them more happy, more productive, or by standing as means to a variety of personally chosen goals which are not strictly job related. As with the first category in which need seemed to play the largest role, this category has fuzzy edges, e.g., treatments that restore one to a functioning capacity spill into both categories. But in the first category, returning one to a functioning capacity may be more job related (i.e., returning one to a functioning capacity makes seeking a job more possible), while functioning capacity in this second category—insurance schemes—allows pursuit of goals that in addition to seeking and holding jobs, may go beyond job-related goals. However, there are still limitations on these other goals, for employment-based insurance typically does not cover treatments such as laser eye surgery that might meet both job-related and other social goals. This discussion of insurance schemes seems to suggest that insurance companies and employers go somewhat further in their health-care coverage than publicly funded schemes, but do not include every conceivable preference for treatments. Since employment-based insurance schemes include a broader spectrum of health care than simply needs in the broad sense, it seems that we, in fact, make a distinction between publicly funded health care and employment-based insurance, and some of these differences lie in the fact that insurance schemes go beyond need in the sense I set out above. Thus, Walzer's claim that an in-depth analysis of our actual practices leads us to interpret the meaning of health care as a need is not supported by this analysis.

There is yet another, fairly obvious, category of health care goods. This category consists of goods such as rhinoplasty, breast enhancement, face lifts, tummy tucks, cryogenics, and other esoteric treatments. Rarely do we find any of these treatments covered by health insurance, and to my knowledge, never are they publicly funded. We could, perhaps, make a distinction between this category and the last by saying that these treatments go beyond contributing to our well-being in some deep sense, but instead satisfy more extravagant tastes, or symbolize success, much as a Mercedes or a Corvette rather than a Ford, symbolizes success in the material world.

In my opinion, the limited availability and provision of these treatments on an 'out-of-pocket' basis, suggests that they are luxury items. And at least at the present time, neither insurance plans nor the voice of the general public as reflected in communally funded health care interpret their social meanings as needs. Thus, again, Walzer's understanding of the meaning of health care as a need is supported only if we ignore the several different kinds of health care, and how they are distributed.

Of course, Walzer may respond to this analysis by saying that my examples are instances of health care being distributed in violation of its deep and inclusive meaning. In other words, he may say that our institutional practices such as underwriting Medicare and Medicaid programs and medical research reflect the decisions the US community has already made with respect to the meaning of health care—that it is a need that should be distributed equally to all citizens. But in my opinion, empirical evidence and a less biased interpretation of the meanings of health care simply do not support that position. We have rather discovered that generally, employment-based insurance provides more coverage than public programs, and that out-of-pocket payments allow even greater coverage than insurance schemes. Moreover, on Walzer's methodology there is nothing more to which we can appeal other than interpretations of practices, traditions, and so on. If we are to distribute goods by their deep and inclusive meanings, then I think the broader the context in which we consider meanings, the more likely we are to discover meanings that give a truer picture of those practices. I might add that it seems highly implausible that we have decided as a nation that certain kinds of treatments such as rhinoplasty and breast enhancement are needs that should be distributed to all who believe they need them.

Principles

In the first chapter, I discussed several different distributive principles. I want to briefly reiterate some of that discussion in the context of our actual health-care practices. I have frequently referred to Walzer's interpretation of health care as a need from which he argues that all health care ought to be distributed by the principle of need. I have also made reference to publicly funded health care as a need. But as I have shown in the last section, the notion of need, by itself, does not distinguish public provision from employment-based provision, for we would be hard-pressed to support the idea that employees do not think of most all of their benefits in their health-care plans as a needed item. In addition, people purchasing their own health care insurance more than likely think of it as a need. Still, we have seen that employment-based and free-market based provision of health care goes beyond that of a need on my construal of the term. Moreover, in some cases, even public provision goes beyond the broad sense of need, e.g., some provision of dental care is included that goes above and beyond that notion. Thus, I do not believe that the notion of need makes the finer grained distinctions that separates any of the prongs of distribution from the others.

I think that in respect to publicly provided health care, Daniels, Green and Walzer are all on the right track; namely, it provides an equal opportunity. Both Daniels and Green claim that health care is important because it protects an equal opportunity to individual life plans. Walzer believes it's important because it protects equal membership status in a community. But I want to spell out the senses in which I mean equal opportunity. First, we might just take "life," in the term "life plans" in a very literal sense, and claim that health care protects life, itself. On this sense, health care protects an equal opportunity to life. Second, we might take the term "life plans," and claim that health care is associated with the ability to pursue jobs or careers. Without health care the underprivileged, unless they are extraordinarily lucky healthwise, cannot compete with the more economically and socially advantaged. Life-threatening diseases and illnesses apparently interfere with the ability to compete, as do many disabilities. In addition, other kinds of what might roughly be called health treatments, such as dental care, are provided under public provision. Some of these dental treatments are provided not so much because of life threats or potential epidemics, but for opportunity reasons. For instance, the loss of front teeth does not interfere much with our ability to eat, but it does interfere with our ability to compete for jobs in a country that places a high value on white teeth and winning smiles. Thus, health care in the public provision goes beyond a broad sense of need, as well, because in addition, it protects an equal opportunity to pursue a career.

There is also a sense in which health care protects equal membership status in a community. Health care has become a massively important good, just as Walzer suggests. Without access to it, people are denied full-membership status in the US. Besides the kinds of treatments listed above, public provision of goods such as prosthetic devices, wheelchairs, crutches, as well as laws providing transportation and access for the handicapped, suggest an equal opportunity (or a more equal opportunity) to participate in the community more fully plays a role in this prong of the distribution. However, I do not see how equal membership status avoids the objection raised to Daniels' account. The justification for health care simply would be too broad. Once we take seriously the plurality of cultures in the US, citizens could claim many kinds of treatment are required to participate in their particular culture. To take one example, Muslims may claim that certain medical treatments are necessary because they will make possible their pilgrimages to Mecca. Once the basic structures of society begin underwriting particular cultural practices, we run the risk of destablizing support for the political framework of society.[4] Thus, I believe that the narrower principle of equal opportunity, i.e., the one that supports jobs and careers, most distinctively underlies and articulates the public provision of health care.

Again, the boundaries between publicly provided health care and employment-based insurance are rather fuzzy. Yet we do see some differences. Insurance schemes typically provide a greater level of health care than provided to Medicaid patients who usually receive less costly (and perhaps less efficacious) treatments for the same kind of illness or disease. More advanced and more costly means of diagnosing illnesses are normally reserved for insurance patients. And Medicaid patients must often wait longer to see a physician, or, as is often the case, they visit emergency rooms more frequently than insurance patients for the treatment of conditions that could easily be handled in a doctor's office. So far as I know, infertility, acne and reconstructive surgery are conditions covered under some insurance schemes, but not under publicly provided funding.[5] Nor are abortions typically covered by public funds. As I have already argued, since practices such as these seem over and above saving lives or posing a public health threat, the difference between them and publicly provided health care seems to lie in wide-spread preferences which improve the well-being of their beneficiaries. At the same time, they are not so extravagant by Western standards as to be thought of as luxury items. And I want to suggest that for several reasons we might think that the principle of merit, or desert, underlies the differences between these two distributions.

First, if an employer provides a more desirable benefit package, she may earn if not the devotion, at least the tendency of employees to remain with her company over a longer period of time. Second, if employees are receiving the treatments for which they have reasonable preferences,[6] they are likely to be happier or more satisfied with their lives. Greater satisfaction, in turn, may well contribute not only to greater profits for an individual company, but also contribute to the economic well-being of the nation. And finally, if employees are more satisfied with their lives they are, I think, more likely to want to offer a hand up to the least advantaged, thus increasing the productivity of the disadvantaged and providing even greater economic benefits to the community (i.e., if improving the lot of the disadvantaged translates into greater opportunities for them). Typically, when benefits are cut back on employees (such as medical care after retirement, or income retirement accounts), it has a tendency to make them become mean-spirited with respect to public funding of welfare programs. But when employees are enjoying good benefits from their companies, they tend to become more magnanimous with the less fortunate. So, in some sense, since the employees not only benefit directly from employment-based insurance, but also contribute to the economic well-being of the nation, we might think that they have earned, or deserve, their greater health-care benefits.

The final category of health care goods—those goods we might call a luxury—also has a corresponding principle of distribution. The free market principle has a long and distinguished history wherever capitalism has gained a stronghold. In Western democracies it expresses the entrepreneurial spirit in which people are free to accumulate and dispose of their legally gained property in any way they wish, so long as they cause no harm to others. If buyers are willing to buy and sellers are willing to sell and no one is harmed or duped and no laws are violated, then citizens are free to carry on their own private affairs without interference from government. In addition, the free market principle expresses the right to use money (the most common medium of exchange) as a means to our individually chosen plans of life. While the free market principle is just one method of distribution, it is, I believe, just as legitimate a representative of distributive principles as those of equal opportunity and merit.

Yet this principle is often rejected by many bioethicists as the proper one under which health care ought to be distributed.[7] I believe their rejection is correct if that were the *only* principle regulating health-care distribution. Health care is not simply a commodity. It is not *simply* any one thing because of its huge variability in services and purposes. However, I see nothing wrong with it in its proper place. If an individual can afford to buy a tummy tuck, a "nose job," breast implants, face lift, and so on, and a seller is willing to sell her services, and no one is harmed, why should we interfere in these practices? Why should there be constraints on these services when we refrain from putting constraints on the kinds of cars we sell? No one thinks we should sell only one kind of car, for that limits people's ability to dispose of their income in ways they wish. So why should we put constraints on the kinds of health care people wish to purchase? These are, after all, *luxury* items, not necessitous items. Admittedly, more expensive treatments may have the effect of driving up the costs of more medically necessary treatments. But that seems more an issue for cost regulation of those treatments rather than an argument for eliminating the freedom to purchase luxury medical items. It thus seems clear that a free market principle governs the upper tier of health care. I see no reason to rule out this kind of provision so long as two constraints are imposed upon it. First, luxury health care items must not negatively interfere with the other two levels by driving up their costs. And second, there are some instances in which certain health care practices are of questionable efficacy, or even may be harmful. The use of laetrile for cancer treatments is such an example. Studies showed that laetrile not only was inefficacious, but that people desperately seeking cures failed to make use of treatments that might have helped them. In light of these findings, the US government banned its use. Since medical technology may be beyond the understanding of many patients, and since many patients are in either a weakened physical or mental state, I believe the government has a legitimate role in protecting its citizens from harm by curtailing medical treatments even when cost is not an issue.

That a case can be made for the three-pronged distribution of health care in this country, i.e., that a three-pronged distribution is more true to our actual practices than the picture Walzer paints, goes some distance in justifying it as the distribution that citizens have actually decided upon. My account, I believe, is a much more accurate interpretation of the meaning of health care, and far less biased, than Walzer's because it takes our actual practices as they *are*, in a wider context, and not as I might *wish* they were. And, as I pointed out in the last chapter, compromise among competing interpretations of justice may very well be at the heart of justice in a pluralistic society. Otherwise put, even if I were biased in favor of an equal distribution of all health care treatments, I believe that I cannot report that *that* is the decision of the US community. To make more firm our convictions that a three-pronged distribution is morally acceptable, in the next section I address issues of methodology and the role of abstraction in decision making.

Methodology, Abstractions, Universalism and Particularism

Walzer is not always clear on the issue of principles. He sometimes speaks as if the meanings of goods generate principles of distribution. "...the principles of justice are themselves pluralistic in form; ... different social goods ought to be distributed for different *reasons*, in accordance with different procedures, by different agents; and ... all these differences derive from different understandings of the social goods themselves..."[8] At other times, he speaks as if there is already a sphere governed by a certain principle, and then we situate a good in that sphere according to its meaning. "Every social good or set of goods constitutes, as it were, a distributive sphere within which only certain criteria and arrangements are appropriate."[9] If we understand Walzer to mean that goods generate principles, then we might think that principles bubble up to the surface from the particular meanings goods possess in a society, thus making the principles, themselves, relative to a society. If we take Walzer to mean that principles with their spheres are already in place and we fill them with certain goods according to their meanings, then that suggests that we already have preconceived notions of these principles. In other words, they do not spring up merely from meanings of concrete goods particular to a society, but from our underlying understandings of principles, as well.

I want to suggest that this second alternative is the case. Walzer argues, for instance, that the social meaning of health care as a *need* puts it in the sphere of communal provision given his understanding of the social contract. Again, his understanding of the social contract is: "it is an agreement to redistribute the resources of the members in accordance with some shared understanding of their needs, subject to ongoing political determination in detail."[10] And in a discussion concerning how justice might be constructed, Walzer says that "it's not only a matter of implementing some singular principle or set of principles in different historical settings ... no one would deny that there is a range of morally permissible implementations."[11] Thus, Walzer first posits a sphere of needs governed by the principle of need, and then locates a good in that sphere if its meaning is that of a need. And the same can be said with respect to his other spheres. Yet, Walzer does not actually tell us where these spheres come from, nor does he argue for these spheres, but simply assumes their existence. Since Walzer fails to discuss how these spheres, themselves, are constructed, they and the principles appropriate to them appear to be no less abstract than Rawls's conception of the person and the role of morality in society from which he derives his distributive principles. It thus seems to me that Walzer and Rawls simply start from different points of abstraction.

So, I do not think we can rid ourselves of the role of abstraction in deciding on just distributions. We, in fact, debate not just about the meanings of social goods, but about the meanings of conceptions of justice. For instance, we debate about the roles the principles of equal opportunity, merit and free enterprise play in the various distributions of goods in our country. How should we understand equal opportunity; how should we understand merit and the market? Are there interrelations between these principles such that, e.g., the marketplace should be constrained by equal opportunity? Thus, principles, themselves, are abstract in nature.

In addition, I think that we should accept that principles are universalistic. Even if we take Marx's economic view, it is not the case that the principle of free enterprise is unknown, but rather that it *is* known, understood, and has been rejected. The principle of equal opportunity may have had its unique history in the US, but it is on that basis which we justify our practice of criticizing nations that fail to recognize it. For instance, even though India's caste system is illegal, it still greatly influences its social practices, and it is on the basis of equal opportunity that we criticize its social practices. Thus, at least in the US, we recognize equal opportunity as a legitimate principle of criticism of other cultural practices. And I believe that it is safe to opine that in virtually every nation, tribe or culture, the principle of merit is responsible for the greater rewards some receive over others. Given this analysis, I want to suggest that the principles underlying all distributions are both abstract and universal in nature, and that at least half the debate about just distributions turns on the meanings of principles in a particular society.

Now Walzer may respond that it is not the universal and abstract nature of principles to which he objects, but rather the attempt to universalize the meanings of goods according to such principles. That is, if a good such as health care is seen as a need in the US and distributed by such a principle, presumably Walzer would say that *that* circumstance does not automatically mean that health care should be distributed by the principle of need in, say, India—it all depends on what health care means in India. And it is *that* which distinguishes his theory from Rawls's. Otherwise put, Walzer argues that the proper starting point is from the meanings of already existing goods, such as "membership, health, food and shelter..."—that is what the main debate is about, and not the meaning of justice. He seems to think that our society is more homogeneous than heterogeneous, and thus it's safe to assume that we all have roughly the same ideas about justice. But that belief is dubious at best. Just in the area of distributive justice, some believe that justice consists in only the free market, and some believe that justice consists in the redistribution of all the wealth. This is actually at odds with his discussion of social goods where he admits controversy about meanings. Why would he think that we debate about the meaning of, say, bread, but not the meaning of justice?

On the other hand, a Rawlsian view takes into account the pluralistic nature of our society, assumes that there is a debate about the meaning of justice, and from there argues for such a conception according to which individual values must be constrained if we are to continue as a stable society. In other words, it takes the main debate to be about the meaning of justice. Of course, Rawls does not simply assume that the meanings of goods are so universal that they can be decided upon in abstraction from particular societies, for he never attempts to set out an exact distribution apart from empirical considerations, but rather leaves that for the legislative stage in the development of institutions (i.e., it becomes a particularistic matter). But Walzer is correct that Rawlsian justice is vague with respect to the distribution of particular goods, and this vagueness makes for indeterminacy in application. Thus, because Walzer starts from a thick theory of social goods, he ignores the debate about justice in a pluralistic nation, and because Rawls starts from a thin theory of goods and focuses on justice, he in effect ignores the debate about particular social goods and their distribution. But neither Rawls nor Walzer can avoid abstractions: Walzer is abstract in his view of spheres and Rawls is abstract in his view of the person situated in a meaningful society who has ideas about concrete social goods.

My analysis of these different starting points thus suggests two consequences: philosophy cannot avoid abstractions—that is its very nature; and second, a rigid adherence to one starting point or another cannot result in a theory that aids policy decisions which are true to *all* our social meanings. We have rough meanings of justice that need to be spelled out and argued for; especially in a pluralistic nation we cannot just assume the meaning of justice. As well, we have rough meanings of goods that need to be spelled out and argued for against the various meanings of justice. My view, then, is that for massively important social goods such as health care, the debate must take place at more than one level: the various meanings of health care must be open for debate, and the various conceptions of justice must be open for debate; neither is a foregone conclusion. Thus, we need to work back and forth between the abstract and the particular, between concepts and concrete goods, in order to establish a coherence between the two. Certainly we want to retain some relativity (though how much is hard to say), for we want our moral practices to make sense to us and reflect the considered decisions we have made as a nation; but at the same time, we must be able to subject shared social meanings of concepts as well as goods, to rational assessment and revision.

Since the actual distribution of health care *is* the three-pronged distribution that I have set out, and since the principles for which I have argued are quite plausibly the ones which govern each of the prongs of distribution, we are now in a position to judge whether our current distribution is just.

Gaps in Health Care Coverage

In this section, I want to refer back to the first chapter. I noted in that chapter several gaps in each of the prongs of our present distribution of health care. I start with publicly funded health care. Figuring conservatively, less than half of the nation's poor are covered by publicly financed health care because they do not qualify. This means that at least 40 million people in the US are not entitled to this social good. Thus, they must either go without it, or the must depend on charity for their health care. Now, if I am correct that the principle underlying this prong of the distribution is equal opportunity, then somewhere around 40 million people are being denied not only the benefit of health care, but if they are ill or disabled, the opportunity to compete for many of the other benefits of society which, themselves, depend on reasonably good health. The ability to compete for most jobs or positions of authority comes immediately to mind. So, as things stand now, this prong of the distribution is in violation of the principle of equal opportunity.

The second prong—employment-based provision—may be understood as a reward for contributing to the economic well-being of the country. Everyone who is employed presumably contributes in some measure to the economy, be that the tax base, or as consumers of manufactured goods, or of services. As contributors to the well-being of the nation, then all who are employed ought to be covered by employment-based health care. Yet, 27.3 to 37.3 percent of the population, or 65 million to 88 million working Americans are underinsured or uninsured (again, these figures are fuzzy). At the beginning of President Clinton's first term in office, part of his health-care plan was to establish that employers must provide health insurance for their employees. Had that plan met with Congressional approval, our nation might now be meeting its responsibilities toward employees. But as we stand now, this prong of the distribution fails to fulfill the obligations set out by the principle underlying it—the principle of merit or contribution.

In respect to the third prong of the distribution—purchasing health care by the ability to pay—there are a couple of ways we might view it. First, we might think that if health-care buyers are willing to spend some amount of money on their health care, and providers are willing to sell it, then the amount of health care buyers receive is fair because they have freely allocated exactly the amount of their budget they wish or need on health care. But on the other hand, we have already seen that some employees (usually low-income ones) do not receive health care insurance, or they are severely underinsured. So, it would be hard to make the case that they are freely making a choice to purchase either no health care, or less health care than they need to supplement their health care package if they have one. Freely making a choice assumes that there are at least two viable options, and that one could have chosen to do otherwise. But clearly low-income workers are unable to exercise an option to buy the amount of health care they need. Nor are many of these people eligible for publicly provided health care because they do not meet federal or state guidelines. Thus, this prong of the distribution fails to provide health care coverage to all its members, just as the other two prongs failed.

Proposal

In this section, I wish to repeat my claim that there is nothing, in principle, wrong with distributing health care according to three, very deeply held values in the US—the principles of free enterprise, merit and equal opportunity. And, in fact, there is a lot to recommend that practice. I think that I need not appeal to one and only one overarching theory from which we might derive a defensible distribution of health care. The many varied and actual uses and meanings of health care work against the notion that there exists one principle, or any one set of principles, from which just distributions arise. Theories are simply too far removed from our actual practices, and ignore, or are unable to take into account, the huge complexities involved in any such distribution. Moreover, the near impossibility of reaching wide agreement on theory, itself, is a stumbling block. Among leading theories such as consequentialism, deontology and virtue ethics, people hold conflicting moral intuitions. Some are thorough-going consequentialists, others thorough-going deontologists, and the same can be said about virtue theory. To add to this, some people hold a deontological view under one circumstance, but a consequentialist view under another, and virtue ethics under still another. Thus the idea that we can depend on only one theory puts an unnecessary strain on our already over-burdened decision-making abilities when decisions about distributions must be decided upon in real time.

Nor do we need to accept our actual practices as just merely because they happen to be the practices we have. That would amount to saying we cannot do better or improve our practices. We can, instead, turn to the principles underlying those practices, using them as criteria to improve our present distribution of health care. Of course, using the underlying principles in this way assumes that they are, indeed, the correct principles that US citizens have decided upon, and that they carry moral weight. But I have already argued that these principles are quite plausible (much more plausible than Walzer's rather single-minded understanding of our health-care practices) because they both express three of our most deeply held values and because they seem to match our intuitions about the many meanings of health care practices in a wider context of understanding.

Thus, the empirical and conceptual evidence for my understanding of both our practices and our principles gives us greater reasons to accept those principles than Walzer's principle of need, or Green's attempt to equate health with the basic liberties, or Daniels's broadened principle of fair equality of opportunity. Moreover, my understanding of health care does not encounter the difficulties that Green's or Daniels's or Walzer's does. It neither comes into conflict with other deeply held values as Green's extension of Rawls's theory does. Nor does it raise questions about how far to extend publicly based provision that Daniels's broadened principle of fair equality of opportunity raises. Nor does it require us to accept the notion that *all* health care is a need, as Walzer's account does. Moreover, since my interpretation covers a broader range of practices than Walzer's, and the principles governing these practices are quite plausibly the principles we have decided upon for the distribution of health care, I propose that we use them as the criteria to develop a more just distribution of the same.

My proposal, then, is to set out a somewhat idealized form of distribution based on the principles of equal opportunity, merit and free exchange. Under the principle of equal opportunity, I propose that everyone who is unemployed and who falls below an income level which either does not allow them to purchase their own insurance, or which makes it necessary for people to trade off one need, for example food and decent housing, for health care, qualifies for public provision of health care. The package for which they would qualify remains indeterminate, but must consist of a decent minimum of health care that would return, restore, or at least improve the functioning capacity of people. The moral justification for this prong of health care is that it provides an equal opportunity for people to pursue careers, when they are unable to provide health care for themselves. This provision suffers from the same questions as Daniels's, Green's, and Walzer's theories: how much and what kind of health care, given scarce resources? But I think that we can give only a rough approximation of a decent minimum, refining and specifying the provision against the idea of equal opportunity and in light of available resources.

Given the principle underlying employment-based provision, all employers must count as part of the cost of doing business, providing health insurance for their employees. Some smaller firms may protest because it is their belief that the costs of insurance are too expensive and will drive them out of business. There are several remedies for that problem. First, in light of the decisions citizens have already made about the provision of health care, I see no reason that federal regulations of the insurance industry should not play a larger role. For smaller firms, health insurance premiums should either be less costly, or smaller firms can band together to obtain coverage at the same rate as larger firms. Second, there should be greater tax advantages for smaller firms. Presumably, smaller firms could write off health care expenses at a greater percentage. Third, if these smaller firms still find insurance too expensive, they may offer employees less income, either per hour or per week (but not below the minimum wage) in exchange for insurance. My guess is that most employees would opt for insurance, but those who wish to opt out, may not qualify for publicly provided health care. The proviso that some may opt out and still not qualify for public provision may indeed be seen as a limitation on some sort of freedom, but these people are free to purchase their own health care if they so desire under the third prong of distribution. Under the employment-based prong, then, all employed people who want it would have health insurance. Again, the actual package is indeterminate, but it, like the publicly provided package, should provide a decent minimum of health care. This leaves companies free to add to a decent minimum in order to compete for employees. Presumably, the better the health care package, the more competition there will be for employment in that firm, and the more likely the firm will establish loyalty from their employees.

The third, and final prong—health care based on free exchange—would simply leave the package of health care to the decision making of the individual purchaser and the provider. This prong would run solely according to how much people are willing to spend and how much providers are willing to sell. Those who previously did not qualify for public provision but were unable to provide their own care would no longer be members of this group. Nor would those who are employed but underinsured or uninsured by their employers. Thus, this prong does not assume that low-income people could have chosen to purchase health care but decided to spend their money on other things. It rather assumes that the members of this group have the income to purchase their own health care or health care insurance. This package of health care is indeterminate too, for people are free to purchase whatever they wish, with one exception. One constraint must, I think, be enforced on this prong: the (presumably) more expensive and more exotic treatments allowed in this category may not be allowed to drive up the costs of either publicly provided or employment provided health care. Again, federal regulations may come into effect here, constraining insurance companies from increasing the costs of coverage for insurance in order to fund the more exotic treatments of the wealthy. This constraint might be seen as an infringement on the freedom to dispose of one's property as one wishes, and an infringement on providers to sell what they wish. But, given our understanding of the various meanings of health care, the constraint is something to which we have already agreed. If the cost of health care is driven up such that we are unable to afford it for the less wealthy, then we have violated the principles underlying the several means of health care distribution. That is, we have violated the implication that everyone's health care is somehow covered.

In the next, and final chapter, I shall set out some troubling cases of health care to see how they might be resolved given this rather idealized version of our existing distribution. I shall refer back to cases such as the differences in treatment between reconstructive surgery and breast enhancement, as well as treatment for lingering neuroses as opposed to mental illnesses, differences in diagnostic procedures, treatment for infertility and abortion and contraceptive measures. I believe that given my proposal, we can find a category into which each of the differences in these treatments might appropriately fit. If the differences in treatments fit appropriately into the different prongs and everyone has access to health care according to the principles underlying each category, then this somewhat idealized version of our present practices is, I believe, defensible.

CHAPTER 6

PRINCIPLES AND APPLICATIONS

In the last chapter, I argued that a somewhat idealized form of our present distribution of health care is defensible if each of the three prongs provides health care according to the principles underlying each prong. Recall that the first level of provision is public funding and the principle underlying this prong, I have argued, is equal opportunity. The second level of provision is employer insurance and its underlying principle is quite plausibly merit or contribution. The third level of provision is provided under the free market principle. I have also argued that differences in treatments should be explained by, or roughly correspond to, these three levels of health care. Thus, when differences in treatments are justified, they are justified only insofar as they make reference to the principles of equal opportunity, merit and free enterprise.

In this chapter I shall set out examples of health care treatments and their availability to members of the three prongs of distribution. Some treatments are, or should be, available to all members of all categories. Some treatments are, or should be, available only to members of the second and third prong. And some treatments are, or should be, available only to members of the third prong. I shall argue that these differences in availability correspond to the three principles underlying each prong. Further, I shall argue that when the treatments required to fulfill the obligations implied by each principle are unavailable to members of these categories, we are in violation of the decisions we have already made with respect to the reasons for supplying health care at each level. This will be especially true at the first level of provision, but may be true of the second level, as well. Otherwise put, the US citizens have at some level of consciousness, already matched principles to treatments and treatments to principles in an attempt to insure that everyone in the US has adequate health care. It is my belief, then, that the fact that our existing distribution is littered with gaps is more accidental than purposeful. The gaps are a result of a failure by government, citizens and health-care providers to make good long-term plans, the fact of the many agencies and providers responsible for health care delivery and the lack of clear directives among these agencies and providers, and—one must admit—the result of some providers who put profits ahead of medically desirable protocols. However, by and large I believe that these accidental (and in some cases purposeful) discrepancies do not reflect the decisions US citizens have made.

I want to start at the communal level of provision for each treatment that I discuss since I think the differences between that and employment-based provision are the most difficult to distinguish and it is here that the greatest disputes arise concerning the fairness of the distributions. But before I begin matching principles to cases, I think a few words need to be said about the equality of opportunity principle and its connection to public provision. I said in Chapter Five that we *might* think that need, construed as providing health care for conditions which either threaten personal or public health or which restore functioning capacity to the extent possible, is the underlying principle. But then I argued that if we think of need in this sense, it does not make the distinction between public provision and employment-based provision that we, in fact, make. Some treatments even at the public level go beyond need in the above sense, e.g., they provide a more equal opportunity to compete for jobs and positions. Nor does the notion of need even make the distinction between public provision and free market provision. For in some sense, all provisions may be thought of as a need (though in my opinion, many of the treatments available on the third level are luxury items). I thus argued that it is the idea of equal opportunity rather than need that sets public provision apart from the other two.

Under my construal of equal opportunity, those who are unemployed and who fall below an income level which makes purchase of certain kinds of health care (or insurance) impossible, or that makes it necessary for them to trade off other important needs for health care, would qualify for public provision. They qualify because without health care, they more than likely will not be in a position to compete for many of the other benefits of society such as places in schools and jobs. Thus, the kinds of health care for which government is obligated are those that repair or alleviate abnormal biological conditions that prevent an equal opportunity for jobs and careers. It seems clear enough, in line with Daniels's account, that the kinds of health care provided at this level would be those that restore, or at least improve the normal functioning capacity of individuals such that these opportunities may be realized. Yet, my account narrows the range of justified claims to health care by reference to positions and careers.

Unlike Daniels, however, I do not include in the idea of equal opportunity a broad sense of "plans of life," meaning life plans that go beyond competition for jobs and careers. His broadened principle of fair equality of opportunity, I believe, leads to too much indeterminacy in application. It is hard to tell what makes the difference between, for instance, a social obligation to provide health care for reconstructive surgery after a mastectomy, but not breast enhancement if we must refer to plans of life in the broad sense that Daniels uses. The same can be said for Walzer's idea of an opportunity to realize equal citizenship status. The idea is simply too broad when we are trying to determine governmental obligations.

My interpretation of equal opportunity, however, does include many of the elderly who are now covered under Medicare simply because upon retirement their income level is substantially reduced and they are not working. The same may be said for those on Medicaid. On the other hand, those who choose to continue working after the age of sixty-five would be covered under employment-based insurance. And those who are unemployed but have a fairly decent income would be covered under the free market.[1] So we need not worry about ageism on my account. That is, health care would not be denied simply on the basis of age; it would not be denied at all. Rather, public provision would be denied to the elderly only if they either have employer insurance or if they are unemployed and can afford it themselves.

Resolution of Troublesome Cases

Let us begin by taking treatments that concern reconstructive surgery after a mastectomy in contrast to breast enhancement. Daniels attempts to include reconstructive surgery under a national health care plan, but exclude breast enhancement by reference to the idea that normal biological functioning (or nearer to normal) is justified by plans of life. But I argued that reconstructive surgery will not return the mastectomy patient to normal functioning, it will only return her to an appearance of normal functioning. And I argued that breast enhancement would make possible a certain plan of life—specifically, a plan related to jobs and careers, while the reconstructive surgery serves only a social function which is unrelated to jobs. What Daniels often fails to make clear is that normal species functioning sets a lower limit on the kinds of health care publicly funded[2] and that lower limit is justified by reference to life plans, broadly construed. So, on the one hand, Daniels attempts to limit social obligations by making use of the notion of normal functioning. But on the other hand, once he goes beyond the traditional sense of life plans (jobs and careers), his account may either obligate society for too much, or it simply causes confusion. We cannot understand, for instance, why including reconstructive surgery is a social obligation, but breast enhancement is not. But I believe that my account can resolve this difficulty.

At the public level of provision neither surgery would be covered, for neither one will return an individual to what we typically mean by normal biological functioning; nor does the lack of either one pose personal or social threats to health. With respect to providing an equal opportunity to compete for jobs, we might think that breast enhancement would more nearly fit this category than reconstructive surgery since larger breasts may make one more eligible to compete for certain jobs. But the same idea applies to reconstructive surgery. Larger, or more perfect, breasts may enhance one's ability to pursue a job or career because they are instances of norms of physical attractiveness in our society. But I think that we need to distinguish between certain norms. The norm of white teeth, for example, applies to everyone in our society, not just females. Moreover, we also understand a full set of teeth and white smiles as an indication of health. But the supposed (sexist?) norm of large breasts applies only to women, and it is by no means clear to me that large breasts are indicators of good health. Hence, since small breasts are not a biological abnormality, and since they seem to be a reflection of sexist societal standards, there is no rationale for such a surgery. That is, they seem to be an irrelevant characteristic in consideration of job placements. Moreover, it does not seem that publicly funded programs should be in the business of promoting sexist stereotypes. Further, the idea of an equal opportunity for jobs does not include competing for specific jobs for which one might have a preference. Rather, it concerns the idea that abnormal biological functioning interferes with seeking jobs, generally. Thus, breast enhancement for the purposes of a seeking a specific job is not justified at the public level. Nor, based on this analysis, does there seem to be a rationale for including reconstructive surgery after a radical mastectomy, since normal functioning cannot be restored and since perfect breasts are an irrelevant consideration.

At the employment-based level of provision, the employer is free to include in a health-care package either of these treatments, although the issue of containing costs is a factor that might work against either of these inclusions. It seems the employer would be more likely to include reconstructive surgery as an added benefit than breast enhancement, perhaps for the same reason we might think that prosthetic devises would likely be included—they give the appearance of normalcy, even if they do not return normal functioning. Obviously, breast enhancement is irrelevant to job performance unless the job is something like an exotic dancer. But why would an employer hire anyone for such a job unless she were already well endowed? However, I see nothing wrong with including that treatment if an employer so desires.

At the highest level of provision—as a commodity—this question almost becomes moot. So long as these treatments do not drive up costs of other treatments for the less well off, I see no reason that people who want it should not be able to purchase it.

In the same area—reconstructive surgery—is the question of whether to include rhinoplasty at different levels of provision. The answer to that question depends on the purpose of the treatment. Treatment for a deviated septum is quite different than molding a nose to fit accepted standards of beauty. If the treatment in question is for a deviated septum, then it seems that both public and employment-based provision must include it, for it interferes with important biological functions such as breathing and sleeping. If the treatment is for molding a nose, I think that public provision in most cases would not include it; for imperfect noses do not interfere with normal biological processes. Nonetheless, I believe that some room must be left open for review of individual cases, for an individual's nose may be so far out of the norm that it would be hard to secure a job. We can grant that this introduces a social stereotype into the discussion and regret the superficiality of society, but numerous studies have shown that appearances have an effect on success in job seeking. This conclusion is consistent with my earlier discussion in Chapter Five concerning the replacement of lost front teeth. While the loss of such does not interfere that much with eating, it does interfere with opportunity.

One may very well ask what the difference is between treatments such as rhinoplasty and breast enhancement; after all, they both concern physical appearances, but neither are necessary for normal biological functioning. First, rhinoplasty is not particular to any one sex—both men and women may be afflicted by extraordinarily unattractive noses. Second, a great deal of the answer may lie in the degree of deviation from the norm, and degree of response to that deviation. Some deviations are far greater and prompt responses of shock, pity and even horror. For people living with that condition, it takes a terrible toll on their self-worth. Thus, their condition not only interferes with opportunity but with mental health. I think the same may be said for burn victims with terrible scars. Their disfigurement not only makes securing a job difficult, but leads to psychological difficulties, neither of which are circumstances for which they are responsible.

In respect to coverage for mental health at the communal provision level, I believe the distinctions between different levels of health care must be made by reference to individual responsibility, abnormal biological brain functioning and how abnormal brain functions interact with or are caused by environmental influences. Many people believe that a sharp line can be drawn between abnormal brain functioning and environmental influences. Yet neurophysiological studies rarely draw any sort of sharp line between the two. Rather, they more often consider biological functioning set against environmental influences. But they think of environmental influences in a rather broad way: in this context, environmental influences include genetic predispositions for a disease, family influences, toxic hazards, and even the environment in which cells develop. For instance, some studies have suggested that when some pregnant women are under a great deal of stress during gestation, intercellular environment may give rise to homosexuality. I do not mean to suggest, here, that homosexuality is an abnormality. My point is rather that neurophysiologists take a larger view on environmental influences on the brain, and importantly, this view entails that individuals are not responsible for their afflictions. It is against this broader view of biological and environmental influences that I want to discuss treatment for mental illnesses. Obviously individuals are not responsible for their genetic make-up, or for environmental influences on the brain. Individuals with diseases such as schizophrenia, bipolar affective disorder, attention deficit disorder, and many forms of depression have a genetic predisposition for developing these conditions. Such diagnoses certainly warrant public provision of treatment. For untreated, those individuals cannot effectively compete on the job market. However, I want to offer a caveat here: if it is deemed they are capable of assuming some responsibility, then once individuals have been diagnosed and treatment ensues, I think they must be in compliance with their treatment in order to receive continuing assistance. One hallmark of mental illness is resistance to treatment for various reasons, but I believe that after some number of chances and agreement among a treatment team that an individual refuses to comply, social obligations come to an end. At some point, the individual must take some responsibility. Of course, if professionals agree that an individual simply cannot take responsibility, then public assistance must continue. For example, people with severe forms of schizophrenia or bipolar disease are so incapacitated by their illness that the idea of taking responsibility is inapplicable.

Most employment-based insurances offer some coverage for mental diseases. I believe that their guidelines for a base should follow public provision. Beyond that, I believe the employer is free to choose. The greater amount of treatments and the greater choice in therapists would obviously act as an incentive to remain with a company. Moreover, return to more normal functioning saves a company the money they have spent on employee training. So, a greater amount of coverage in mental health care may be expected since those treatments contribute to overall economic well-being to which employees have contributed.[3]

At the free market level, again, the question is almost moot. People are free to choose the kinds and amounts of therapy offered on the free market. One cautionary word here: As with many areas of medicine, there are some experimental, even highly controversial forms of treatment.[4] Just because a patient has the means with which to purchase any treatment she or he may wish, I believe that the government nonetheless has a duty to protect its citizens from harmful procedures. This is especially true when people are in a weakened physical state or susceptible mental state. Thus, we would expect some sort of governmental safeguards even under circumstances in which people can afford whatever they wish. To be sure, governmental safeguards are paternalistic. But I think they are not unjustified paternalism if an individual simply is not in a condition to make decisions in their own best interests.

I think it is best to treat infertility as an issue distinct from abortion and contraceptive measures. Infertility concerns issues of abnormal biological function, while abortion and contraception do not. Clearly, the inability to have children has social implications as well—one may be seen as less of a woman or man if one is unable to produce offspring, perhaps just because the inability is biologically unusual. Still, I do not believe that it is a treatment that should be covered under public funding, nor has it been decided by the community that it should be. I think the best way to approach this issue is to remember, first, the moral justification for health care under this prong: it is ultimately to secure equal opportunity for jobs. Second, that rationale is the justification for types of health care which treat biological abnormalities only insofar as those abnormalities or impairments affect the ability to pursue jobs and careers. Thus, just because an individual has some biological impairment, it does not follow that she or he is entitled to just any publicly funded health care. Since infertility does not affect the ability to pursue careers, then treatment for it is not justified under public provision.[5]

Under employment-based provision, infertility treatments may be covered. Conceiving a child may make an individual happier and be in line with her individually chosen goals; however, I do not see that treatment for infertility is a requirement of employment insurance. My understanding of this sort of treatment is that it is quite expensive. Due to that expense, it may drive the costs of insurance beyond what is reasonable to believe an employer is obligated, and it may very well preclude treatments that apply to all, or most all, employees for which they have a reasonable preference. However, if an employer wishes to include this in a package of benefits, and that inclusion does not affect more basic treatments, I see no reason not to do it. Again, at the third level of provision, the question of infertility treatments seems almost moot. The only constraint on them would be that they do not increase the costs of medical care such that public provision and employer's health insurance coverage becomes too expensive for them.

I want to treat contraceptive measures and abortion together. I believe that both of these treatments should be included in a public package of health care benefits. Yet, neither contraceptive devices nor therapeutic abortions are covered under Medicaid. I think one way to approach contraceptive devices is to first make a distinction between natural and normal biological states. For fertile women, pregnancy may be the natural outcome of sexual intercourse. But then, getting the flu may be the natural outcome of being exposed to a virus.[6] It seems uncontroversial that preventive treatment for the flu should be covered under public funding, yet pregnancy prevention may be more controversial. I want to suggest first, that there are religious differences between pregnancy prevention and flu prevention. Roman Catholics, at least officially, object to contraceptive devices. For the most part, these objections are based on natural law. Yet, I believe that natural-law arguments are extremely slippery, since the notion of "natural" is itself slippery.[7] Moreover, if intervention in natural processes (whatever that means) were the only grounds upon which one is arguing, then lots of interventions would be forbidden. For instance, using life-saving devices would be forbidden by Roman Catholic physicians and patients since those interfere in the natural dying process. But Roman Catholics do not object to using life-saving devices. So, arguments based upon the notion of "natural" cannot stand alone—they require a further premise. Typically, that further premise is based on the Biblical injunction "to be fruitful and multiply." And behind that injunction was the issue of under-population in an age that is far behind us. We are now much more concerned about overpopulation. Thus, originally, the command to be fruitful and multiply was important for the continuation of the race (more specifically, for the continuation of a people who practiced a certain religious faith). I expect we could go so far as to say that being fruitful and multiplying was required for the biological continuation of people of a certain religious faith. Now, however, the biological continuation of the race, itself, is dependent on curtailing reproductive capacity. So, I suppose that in some sense, we could say that contraceptive measures prevent a public health threat since overpopulation can lead to, e.g., food shortages and other problems which negatively effect public health. Thus, contraceptive devices should be part of the package of public funding.

In addition, since pregnancy may interfere with an equal opportunity for jobs, especially for women with low incomes, we find a second reason to fund contraception. It might be objected that since pregnancy is a *natural* outcome of sex (i.e., it is not surprising given our biological make-up), that contraception should not be funded. It is true that pregnancy is a natural outcome of sexual intercourse, but I have already argued that the notion of "naturalness" cannot carry the argument. Nor do I believe that pregnancy is a *normal* condition; and by "normal" I mean "customary" or "usual." From the time women are first able to conceive until menopause, most of that time women are not pregnant. And once a woman first learns she is pregnant, she typically does not believe that she is in a "normal" biological condition. She rather believes that she is in a non-normal biological condition, a belief that is born out by biological and psychological changes. She may experience biological responses such as morning sickness, fatigue, cramping, anemia, and heartburn among other symptoms. She experiences obvious major bodily changes. She also may be subject to minor or major mood swings accompanying hormonal changes. Moreover, the health care community emphasizes the belief that pregnancy is a non-normal state in its admonitions to seek medical care when women first suspect that they are pregnant, much as it admonishes people to seek medical care when they first suspect they might have cancer. So even if it is argued that pregnancy is a natural result of sexual intercourse, it is nonetheless not a normal biological state in the sense of normal that I have defined. Thus, either on threats to public health grounds, or on threats to individual normal biological conditions, I believe that contraceptive measures are justifiable on the first level of health-care provision.

I believe that the argument supporting contraceptive devices on the public level has as much force on the employer level. Typically, insurance schemes do not cover contraceptives, although there have been moves in California for just such coverage.[8] On the part of insurance companies, the idea seems to be that contraceptives are optional for women, and so they need not be covered. Aside from the fact that women then pay more out-of-pocket expenses for their medical needs than men, clearly this scheme interferes with plans of life both in respect to maintaining jobs and pursuing promotions, and in respect to other social goals for which women might have reasonable preferences. Moreover, as I argued earlier, we are much more concerned with overpopulation rather than under-population now. This is a concern not just for women, but for all people. Thus, it seems quite unclear why only women are burdened with the costs for which we all ought to be concerned. So, on the scheme of distribution that I have set out, contraceptive devices ought to be covered at the employment level and failure to do so is in violation of that scheme.

Non-therapeutic abortions are normally not publicly funded either, basically because they are not seen as a health-care need. Since normal pregnancies fail to qualify as ill health, it seems that non-therapeutic abortions cannot be included in publicly funded provision. I think, however, that the same arguments can be advanced to support abortion as were advanced to support contraceptive measures. That is, if pregnancy is not a *normal* condition, and it interferes with a woman's ability to seek a job and work outside the home, then within certain limits I believe that it is justified. It is especially true that unwanted pregnancies among poor women interfere as much in their ability to pursue careers as any physical or mental illness. Moreover, women who either have abortion covered under employment-based or private insurance have an advantage in pursuing their careers over poor women who do not have the resources for an abortion should they want one. First, the better off can afford childcare so that they can continue on their jobs. Second, the less well off are already disadvantaged; an inability to obtain desired abortions would simply make them even worse off. Thus, even if we want to insist that pregnancy is a normal state, it seems there is reason enough to include abortions in the public package of health care. I would think, however, that unless there are health reasons at stake, abortion should not be allowed after the third trimester since it may very well have the affect of undermining our respect for human life.[9]

Another controversial area of medical treatments concerns the issue of life-saving devices and measures. For instance, they include devices such as ventilators that make possible continued respiration and heart beat when patients would otherwise die from illness or injury. And they include measures such as cardiac pulmonary resuscitation when an individual has quit breathing. Whether these devices and measures should be covered under any of the levels of health care provision would depend, I should think, on the probable outcomes to the patient, and on whether they interfere with other provisions deemed more efficacious at the public and employer levels. In addition, I believe that there is another consideration with respect to life-saving devices; namely, that the state has an interest in protecting innocent lives. Hence, any public provision of health care made by the state should not be in conflict with the legal decisions it has made. Consider the following case in which a series of dilemmas present themselves.

Dority v. Superior Court of San Bernardino County is a case in which the legal issue was whether judicial intervention regarding the termination of life support systems was proper.[10] On November 16, 1982, Kristopher DeWayne Dority, a 19-day-old infant, was brought to the emergency room of a hospital by his parents, and later tranferred to Loma Linda University Medical Center (LLUMC). The infant's parents brought him to the hospital after noticing an "odd twitching activity of the left arm which doctors interpreted as a seizure disorder." Diagnostic procedures indicated increased intercranial pressure. The treatment for this condition is decreasing the amount of carbon dioxide in the blood, a procedure that is done by increasing respirations. Since the infant was already experiencing irregular and shallow respirations, the doctors placed him on a respirator. The infant's condition, however, continued to deteriorate. Within a week he failed to respond to any stimulation. Electroencephalograms and cerebral blood flow tests were ordered to determine the viability of the brain.[11] These tests showed electrocerebral silence, which means little, if any, electrical activity in the brain. Testing was performed again about one month later with the same results. The doctors determined that the infant was brain dead.[12] As a result of this diagnosis, removal from life support was recommended.

Normally in these circumstances, LLUMC has a policy of including the parents in the decisionmaking process as to when the child should be removed from life support. These circumstances, however, were not normal. The admitting physician while making a medical background check, had reason to suspect that child abuse had led to the infant's condition. He then reported this circumstance to the proper authorities. Thus, at the time of the recommendation for removal of life support, the parents were being held on charges of felony child neglect or child abuse. Since the parents on the advice of counsel withheld consent to withdraw, the hospital petitioned the court to appoint a guardian for Kristopher in "order to secure consent of a responsible person to terminate the life-support device."[13] The court appointed The Director of the Department of Public Social Services as temporary guardian who sought court guidance as to how he should proceed. The court found that the hospital had used proper medical procedures to determine brain death in this case, and that the medical diagnosis was unrefuted by any medical experts. It thus ordered the temporary guardian to give consent to LLUMC to withdraw the life support system from Kristopher.

Both the parents and counsel for the infant, however, petitioned the appellate court for a writ of prohibition against removing the life-support device on the grounds that judicial intervention was improper in assigning a temporary guardian to act in the best interests of the infant and in ordering withdrawal of life-support devices. Before the court could make a ruling in this case, the child's bodily functions ceased and the life-support device was removed.

The court nonetheless argued that they should render an opinion in this case, since it involved issues of "continuing public interest [that] are likely to recur in other cases."[14] The basis in California upon which withdrawal of life-support devices was established was the Natural Death Act, which acknowledges in adults the right to control decisions relating to the rendering of their own medical decisions.[15] "More specifically, section 7186 [of the Health and Safety Code] 'recognizes the right of an adult person to make a written directive instructing his physicians to withhold or withdraw life-sustaining procedures in the event of a terminal condition'"[16] And in other jurisdictions, this right is thought to be "an expression of the sanctity of individual free choice and self-determination as fundamental constituents of life ... [that] is threatened by the failure to allow a competent human being the right of choice."[17] In the *Dority* case, the court reasoned that if it is legally permissible to refuse or withdraw treatment from a patient who is not yet brain dead, then it is *a fortiori* permissible for a guardian acting in the best interests of the infant to consent to withdrawing treatment from a patient who *is* brain dead. The court also held that while hospitals or physicians do not need to get a court order to withdraw life-support devices in the typical brain-death case, in a contested case it is prudent, since both the health care providers and the guardian might be open to criminal or civil liability. Hence, the appellate court found that the trial court's intervention was appropriate, and on that basis, refused to grant the writ of prohibition to withdraw life support.

The decisions made in the *Dority* case made clear that where there exists no conflict between interested parties, and where proper medical procedures and diagnoses are observed, there are no civil or criminal liabilities attached to discontinuation of life-support systems. The analysis of the *Dority* case does not make clear, however, when patients are entitled *to* life-support systems. Presumably, doctors who do not order life-support when it is a medically appropriate and customary practice, can be held liable for malpractice. If doctors could be held liable for non-treatment with life support when it is appropriate, then it would seem that life support should be included in publicly funded health care. We can hardly expect physicians to parcel out inconsistent treatment according to different health-care plans, or non-existent plans when it may put them in legal jeopardy. Hence, it seems that life-support treatment would be a required element of a publicly funded health care package.

Still, these treatments can be quite expensive; thus the extent to which it should be offered is an issue. In accordance to the principle underlying public provision, it seems that once it has been determined by a treatment team that a patient is irreversibly brain dead, treatment should be discontinued simply because there is no hope of improving an individual's chances for pursuing careers. Moreover, continuation of life support in a case like this would most certainly result in an unequal distribution of scarce resources that cannot be justified by appeal to equal opportunity. On the other hand, if diagnostic procedures indicate hope for some recovery, then we would expect to see continued life-support treatment. It's difficult to say how much recovery warrants continued treatment; but I suppose that many factors exist for such a decision. For instance, if the patient has signed an advanced directive stating the conditions under which she or he does not wish continued treatment that must be counted in the equation. Also, I think we would do well to remember the commitment we have to respecting life. Neither the medical community nor the US community as a whole wants to be in the business of prematurely removing patients from life support when there is hope for recovery.

I wish to discuss another case that has implications for all three prongs of the distribution. Consider the case of Mrs. Helga Wanglie, an

85-year-old patient in a persistent vegetative state (PVS), who was on a respirator.[18] Doctors were in agreement that she received no benefit from such treatment and recommended the respirator be withdrawn. Her husband, however, insisted on continued treatment on the grounds that "We felt that when she was ready to go that the good Lord would call her."[19] After more than a year, and several court actions, Mrs. Wanglie died of multisystem organ failure as a result of septicemia while still on the respirator. The hospital involved in this case had sought legal advice since it did not know its legal obligations. No one in this case knew with certainty Mrs. Wanglie's thoughts about continued life support while in a PVS, so the most that could be done was appoint a conservator to act in her best interests. Thus, one legal action the hospital took was to request that the court appoint an independent conservator to determine whether the respirator was benefiting the patient. The court appointed Mr. Wanglie, an attorney himself, as his wife's conservator. And her conservator, Mr. Wanglie, thought that the timing of Mrs. Wanglie's death should be in the hands of God.

At the beginning of this discussion concerning the Wanglie case, I said it had implications for all three prongs of the distribution. Her health care costs were covered by both Medicare and private insurance. But the question is, Just because she had both Medicare and private insurance, ought this expensive treatment been allowed to continue? At the public level of provision, I think not. For her treatment could not improve her chances for jobs, nor would removal from life-support threaten her life since she was already brain-dead—i.e.—she only gave the appearance of being alive. She had been correctly diagnosed in a PVS and eventually died from her illness. To insist on continued treatment under these circumstances simply consumes public resources that are already scarce and could be put to better use.

Nor do I believe private insurance should have covered her care in this circumstance. Some kinds of treatments covered by private insurance do not have much effect on either the public or the employer distributions of health care. For example, many cosmetic treatments or cryogenic treatments take place in private hospitals or clinics. Thus, the whole constellation of the medical care lies outside of facilities that care for both privately and publicly funded patients. But Mrs. Wanglie's treatment took place in two public facilities: Hennepin County Medical Center and a chronic care hospital. These are the sorts of facilities that are largely publicly funded and it is precisely these kinds of medical care that consume scare resources (including nursing personnel). And it should be noted that part of the reason for increased health-care costs can be traced to insurance plans which allow that portion of the population who can afford them to drive up the costs of health care for everyone else. Thus, the stipulation that expensive treatments that effect public and employer coverage should constrain treatments such as these.

The above case, and the following case are normally termed cases of medical futility. That is, there is little to no hope that treatment can return an individual to anything like normal functioning, nor can it even improve the chances of individuals living an impaired existence. The Lakeberg twins were born sharing a single heart, a single liver and with multiple congenital abnormalities.[20] In order to separate the twins, one had to be sacrificed and medical experts gave the remaining twin a one percent chance of survival from the surgery. In addition, even if one should survive the surgery, her chances of surviving to childhood were remote, much less living any sort of normal life. Their parents, Kenneth and Reitha Lakeberg, nonetheless insisted that surgery be performed even though they had no medical insurance. Against all odds, one of the twins (Angela) did survive the surgery. Most of her treatment occurred at Children's Hospital of Pennsylvania in Philadelphia, with the state of Indiana paying $1000 per day toward the cost of her care, and Children's Hospital absorbing the rest. The total bill for the surviving twin exceeded $1 million at Children's Hospital alone. Angela left the hospital after six weeks, but not to go home. Rather, she was transferred to another public facility where she remained ventilator-dependent until she died, without her parents by her side, just short of her first birthday. Her mother was living with her parents in Indiana, and her father was incarcerated on theft charges. In every respect, this case is a tragedy around which many moral issues arise. But the main question, here, is whether this sort of treatment should be publicly funded, covered by employer insurance, or privately funded.

At the level of public funding, I do not see how the surgery could be justified under the equal opportunity principle. The chances for survival were almost nil; as well, the chances for an opportunity to compete for jobs were as remote. It may seem harsh to make such an indictment, but I believe that hard decisions are part of the equation in publicly funded treatments. We otherwise run the risk of health care being the "bottomless pit" that Charles Fried recognizes it could be.[21] His view is that once we allow the idea of opportunity as a justification for health care, that national health care expenses will be so enormous they will consume the ends at which we aim. For instance, if we spend so much on health care, we will not be able to afford higher education that makes possible our ability to compete on the world market. Without the ability to compete on the world market, businesses may very well fail and the opportunities accruing to those business may very well fail, as well. Thus, not just any opportunity at all costs can justify the kinds of expenses seen in the Lakeberg case. There must exist a reasonable chance that the patient can even survive to realize an opportunity. So, on the one hand, Fried is correct that publicly funding health care on the basis of equal opportunity may have negative effects on overall opportunity. But on the other, health care is importantly related to equal opportunity. The strategy is not to do away with it as a justification, but rather, to insure that equal opportunity is not so broadly construed as to interfere with other provisions that support it. Thus, the equal opportunity principle does not justify publicly funded treatments such as were found in this case.

Nor do I believe the principle of merit can justify this sort of treatment. First, the surviving twin had not met the qualification of merit, i.e., she had done nothing to deserve more advanced treatment than could be expected at the public level. Second, her parents were unemployed, so not even by extension to their children does the principle of merit qualify the twin for this expensive treatment. Again, this may sound harsh. But, again, I believe that treatments of this sort, were they allowed, would make coverage of other, more efficacious treatments much harder to provide.

One might think that at the private level of provision this sort of treatment would be allowed. For free market principles seem to justify spending money any way one wishes so long as no one is harmed or misled. However, I have stipulated a constraint on this provision: medical care that drives up the costs for everyone else should be regulated, and if under regulation it still interferes with provision at the lower two levels, then it cannot be allowed. I believe that even if futile cases such as the Lakeberg twins' were regulated, their costs would still be excessive. Moreover, like the Wanglie case, use of public facilities entails inordinate use of publicly funded research and training as well as nursing and other staff who could otherwise spend their time with patients who are much more likely to benefit from care.

In the area of diagnostic protocols, we also see differences among the prongs of distribution. Typically, those who are publicly provided for receive less sophisticated diagnostic tests, while those at the middle and upper level receive increasingly sophisticated tests. For example, magnetic resonance imaging (MRI) diagnostics normally are not included at the public level, but may be included at the employment level, and of course are available at the private level. MRIs are superior over, for instance, computerized tomograpy (CT) scans and traditional x-ray procedures in diagnosing certain illnesses that involve soft tissue, such as cancer. Referring to the different principles underlying the distribution of health care, if an MRI does a better job diagnosing a condition, and if there is a reasonable hope that diagnosis and treatment will return normal functioning to an individual, then MRIs should be covered under public funding. This sort of decision should crucially involve the attending physician, for she is probably in a better position to decide whether an MRI (a more expensive diagnostic tool than either CT scans or x-rays) is warranted.

Again, I believe that publicly funded medical care should set the baseline for employment insurance. If a condition can be better diagnosed with an MRI, then MRIs should be used rather than CT scans or x-rays. If MRIs are only marginally better in diagnosing a condition, then I suppose they would nonetheless be justified under employer insurance. Employers and insurance companies should be cautious about over-use of this tool, though, just because of its expense. A single MRI series can easily cost $1000. If an MRI has no advantages over, for instance, traditional x-rays—diagnosing a broken bone comes to mind here—then in the interests of saving costs, it should not be used. I think the same line of reasoning applies to private insurance. If an MRI offers no diagnostic benefits, then it should not be used, for the costs of such treatments may have a ripple effect on public and employment medical care.

The conclusion that more expensive diagnostics such as MRIs should be used at the public level if they are medically warranted, is in line with some recent decisions made with respect to health maintenance organizations (HMOs) and Medicare patients. Senior citizens on Medicare are increasingly encouraged to use HMOs for their health care.

Recently the denial of certain services to senior citizens has been the subject of appeal. Helen Alkire's doctor ordered a bone density scan to check for bone damage from osteoporosis.[22] Aetna, Alkire's Medicare HMO refused the test. Alkire appealed the case to Network Design Group, a New York consultant firm that handles appeals for the federal government. Months later, Aetna Senior Choice was ordered to give Alkire the test. Thus, it appears that if a treatment is diagnostically efficacious it should be offered at the public level of distribution.

I could go on at length about different treatments and their availability at different levels of health care. But I believe a picture is emerging from this discussion that justifies my scheme of health care delivery. Health care is not a homogeneous good; it rather serves different purposes and functions, and those different purposes and functions are captured by the principles underlying each prong of our existing distribution. Of course there is a strong component of the idea of need in each distribution, but I do not believe that this idea distinguishes one prong of the distribution from the others. I do believe, however, that the principles of opportunity, merit or contribution, and the free market not only are the underlying principles of each prong, but would serve quite well as the criteria for judging the justice of each prong, and for the distribution of health care in its entirety.

The problem of health care distribution lies not in its principles, but rather in its failure to fulfill the obligations entailed by its principles. Thus, rather than seeking a singular principle under which to unify health care distribution, I believe our efforts should be directed toward insuring that everyone's health care is met in accordance with the three-pronged scheme that I have laid out. This conclusion may be disappointing to some who would like to see, e.g., a single-payer plan of health care in which everyone is entitled to the same access to all available treatments. But the arguments presented here simply do not support that idea. Many forms of health care, e.g., many cosmetic treatments, cannot be defended at the level of public provision; nor can even all life-saving care be justified at that level. Health care, I believe, is a unique good that cannot easily fit under any one principle. Rather, because of its complexity, formulations for its just distribution must be more inventive. We can (and do, I have argued) rely on universal principles as criteria for health care distribution, but its complexity requires creative and innovative ways of putting these principles together in a coherent whole. It requires an open-mindedness to think of health care in its many aspects, and certainly a willingness to compromise between competing ideas of justice. We are a pluralistic nation, and we are dealing with a pluralistic good. In virtue of that pluralism, I believe that approaching a just distribution of health care must come from as many angles as are profitable. It may be the case that some areas of philosophy can afford to do analyses about an issue without much consideration of empirical data. But I believe that I have shown that using only that method does not work in at least one area of applied philosophy; namely, in the area of health care delivery.

I do not know whether the scheme that I have set out is even generalizable to distributions of other tangible or non-tangible social goods. Certainly we would not want a hierarchy of liberties and freedoms. I agree with Rawls that the scheme I have set out is at the wrong level for the basic structures of society. The three-pronged scheme might be generalizable to more tangible goods. But because of the uniqueness of health care, I do not claim that this scheme would work, nor does any tangible good come immediately to mind that might fit into this scheme.

I think that the most important thing to keep in mind, is not that we find a "perfect" scheme of health-care delivery that neatly unifies health care under one principle. But rather, that we find a defensible scheme that insures health care for all US citizens whether they are young, old, productive, poor or wealthy. It is no longer plausible to deny the importance of health care in our country to all citizens. The only plausible questions concern its just distribution. I believe my plan is both just, and justifiable to everyone who is affected by health-care policy. To even continue thinking of our nation as a state that values justice tempered by compassion, we cannot provide health care to only some while others suffer in various ways from its lack. For otherwise, we run the risk of allowing out nation to become something abhorrent to ourselves. I wish to conclude this dissertation by quoting Hubert Humphrey, who, I believe, said in a capsule what has taken me so long to say:

> It was once said that the moral test of government is how that government treats those who are in the dawn of life, the children; those who are in the twilight of life, the elderly; and those who are in the shadows of life, the sick, the needy and the handicapped.[23]

NOTES

Chapter 1

1. Ronald Green, "Health Care and Justice in Contract Theory Perspective," in *Ethics and Health Policy*, eds. Robert Veatch and Roy Branson (Cambridge, Mass.: Ballinger, 1976).

2. Norman Daniels, *Just Health Care* (Cambridge, Mass.: Cambridge University Press, 1985).

3. John Rawls, *A Theory of Justice* (Cambridge, Mass.: The Belknap Press of Harvard University Press, 1971).

4. Michael Walzer, *Spheres of Justice* (Basic Books, 1983).

5. Source: Health Care Financing Administration: Data from the Office of National Health Statistics. Office of Personal Management.

6. Of course some employers provide no health care insurance at all. This issue will be addressed later.

7. The Twentieth Century Fund, *Medicare Reform: A Twentieth Century Fund Guide to the Issues* (New York: Twentieth Century Fund Press,1995).

8. According to *Compton's Interactive Encyclopedia.*, social-insurance programs differ from welfare programs in several respects. Social insurance has the following characteristics: (1) Participation is compulsory. Everyone, including children age 5 or older, is required to

have a Social Security number. (2) Eligibility for benefits and levels of benefits depends on past contributions made by wage earners. (3) Benefit payments begin at a stipulated time such as at retirement from work, upon temporary unemployment, or with disability. (4) Unlike welfare programs, social-insurance benefits are not means-tested, one's wealth or lack of it does not determine whether benefits are granted.

9. The Twentieth Century Fund, *Medicare Reform: A Twentieth Century Fund Guide to the Issues* (New York: Twentieth Century Fund Press, 1995).

10. Ibid.

11. Medigap is private insurance purchased by Medicare beneficiaries to cover many of the costs that Medicare does not.

12. The Twentieth Century Fund.

13. The Twentieth Century Fund.

14. On August 22, 1996, President Clinton signed The Personal Responsibility and Work Opportunity Act of 1996 [H.R. 3734] which reverses a federal guarantee to the poor that has existed since the New Deal days of President Franklin Roosevelt.

15. Medicare coverage for the wealthy may have the effect of reducing the available funds for people outside the high income group.

16. Joel Weissman, "Uncompensated Hospital Care," in *The Journal of the American Medical Association*, September 11, 1996, vol. 276, No. 10, p. 823.

17. Press Enterprise, A1, July 21, 1996.

18. Weissman, "Uncompensated Hospital Care," in *Journal of the American Medical Association*, September 11, 1996, Vol. 276, No. 10, p. 823. These figures are difficult to estimate because there is no commonly accepted definition of underinsurance.

19. J.S. Weissman, Lukas C. Van Deusen, A.M. Epstein, "Bad Debt and Free Care in Massachusetts Hospitals: The Role of Uninsured and Underinsured Patients," in *Health Affairs*, Summer 1992; 11:148-161.

R.J. Blendon, K. Donelan, C.A. Hill, W. Carter, D. Beatrice, D. Altman, "Paying Medical Bills in the United States: Why Health Insurance Isn't Enough," *The Journal of the American Medical Association*, 1994; 271:949-951. Health Resources and Services Administration. *The Hill-Burton Uncompensated Services Program: A Profile*. Rockville, Md: Health Resources and Services Administration; 1994.

20. This statistic is cited from estimates made by the Urban Institute in a press release made by the American College of Physicians, Philadelphia, October 23, 1995.

21. Eric Banfield, *A Heartland Perspective: The Folly of Employer-Based Health Insurance*, The Heartland Institute (Westmont, IL), August 17, 1994.

22. Michael Walzer, *Spheres of Justice*, (Basic Books, Inc.), 1983.

23. Bernard Williams, "The Idea of Equality," pp 240-241.

24. 35 percent of doctors limit their participation in Medicaid, and 5 percent accept no new patients; only 34 percent have full participation.

Chapter 2

1. John Rawls, *A Theory of Justice* (Cambridge, MA: The Belknap Press of Harvard University Press, 1971).

2. Ronald M. Green, "Health Care and Justice in Contract Theory Perspective," in *Ethics and Health Policy*, eds. R. Veatch and R. Branson (Cambridge, MA: Ballinger, 1976).

3. Rawls, p. 19.

4. Ibid., p. 88.

5. Ibid., p.544.

6. Green (1976), p. 116.

7. Ibid., p. 117.

8. Ibid., p. 117.

9. Ibid., p. 117.

10. Ibid., p. 117.

11. Ibid., p. 112.

12. Ibid., p. 117.

13. John Rawls, *Political Liberalism* (New York: Columbia University Press, 1993).

14. Ibid., p. xxv.

15. I shall adopt Rawls's strategy when making references to *A Theory of Justice*, and simply italicize the word "theory."

16. Rawls, *Political Liberalism*, p. 19.

17. Ibid., p. 19.

18. Ibid., p. 106.

19. In fact, Christian Scientists do not believe that even the members of their own faith must forego medical care. Rather, they simply "maintain their right to rely on non-medical health care through spiritual means alone for themselves and their children. The choice of a health care system, however, is always left up to the individual Christian Scientist . . . (moreover) Christian Scientists are bidden to follow the Golden Rule and would not try to impose their beliefs regarding health care on others. They would expect those of other faiths to choose the health care system they trust, and, unless asked, would consider it inappropriate to proselytize." Personal e-mail communication from the manager at The Church of Christ, Scientist, March 26, 1998.

20. Green (1976), p. 117.

21. Ibid., p. 118.

22. Rawls (1971), p. 542-3.

23. Ibid., p. 543.

24. Green (1976), p. 117.

25. Ibid., p. 112.

26. Ibid. , p. 121.

27. Ibid., p. 120.

28. Ibid., p. 117.

29. Hugo Adam Bedau argues this point in "Capital Punishment, Retributive Justice, and Social Defense," in *Moral Controversies*, Steven Jay Gold, ed. (Belmont, CA: Wadsworth Publishing), pp. 237-254

30. This assumption seems to be fairly reasonable since we are in the first place dealing with a distributive theory that takes as fundamental that social resources are limited to some degree.

31. The idea of lexical priority of principles assumes the special conception of justice. I am supposing that Green means this conception since he does not distinguish between the general and the special conception and since he all along talks about the priority of the equal liberty principle over the second principle. It should also be remembered that Green characterizes his principle as a general principle, and not one that is derived from either of the two principles of justice.

32. Rawls (1971), p. 101.

33. Ibid.

34. John Rawls, "Social Unity and Primary Goods," in *Utilitarianism and Beyond*, eds., A. Sen and B. Williams (Cambridge, MA: Cambridge University Press, 1982), p. 168.

35. Ibid., p. 168.

Chapter 3

1. In fact, this is the project Frank Michelman sets for himself in "Constitutional Welfare Rights and *A Theory of Justice*," in *Reading Rawls*, ed. Norman Daniels (Stanford University Press, 1989).

2. Rawls tends to use the term "legitimate expectation" in place of rights. Legitimate expectations, then, are rights and claims based on those rights that arise in accordance with the rules of the social system.

3. Norman Daniels, *Just Health Care* (Cambridge, MA: Cambridge University Press, 1985).

4. David Braybrooke, "Let Needs Diminish that Preferences May Prosper, in *Studies in Moral Philosophy* American Philosophical Quarterly Monograph Series, No. 1 (Oxford: Blackwells, 1968). In Daniels, p. 26. Some of the needs on this list are obviously problematic if we understand them to be needs for which society is responsible. Take the example of a mate in one's prime. In personal communication with Daniels, he does subscribe to the idea that "we have obligations to address departures from normal functioning that make it difficult or impossible for people to sustain the kind of relationship needed to have a mate." However, he disavows accepting at face value all the needs on this list. I think rather that this list is meant to give us a general idea of the sorts of needs which are objectively ascribable, but not necessarily ones for which society is responsible (at least not without some fairly careful argumentation). E-mail communication, 1/18/97.

5. J. H. McCloskey, "Human Needs, Rights, and Political Values," *American Philosophical Quarterly*, 13:1. In Daniels, p. 26.

6. Ibid., p. 17.

7. Ibid., p. 27.

8. Ibid., p. 28.

9. Ibid., p. 28.

10. Ibid., p. 43.

11. Sometimes Rawls's principles are spoken of in shorthand, with the first principle called the liberty principle and the second called the equality principle. Daniels insists that his theory of health care does not necessarily depend on Rawls's theory. On the other hand, his theory depends crucially on the elements of Rawls's theory that are most notable. For instance, Daniels claims that *if* Rawls's version of equal opportunity is justified, then so is a social obligation to provide health care.

12. Rawls, "Social Unity and the Primary Goods," in *Utilitarianism and Beyond*, eds. A.K. Sen and B. Williams (Cambridge University Press, 1982), p. 168.

13. Will Kymlicka makes a similar point in *Contemporary Political Philosophy* (New York: Oxford University Press, 1990), pp. 70-73.

14. Ibid., p. 41.

15. Ibid., p. 104.

16. Ibid., p. 103.

17. Ibid., p. 28.

18. This account of biological functioning and its effect on mental states leaves open the question of whether either environmentally caused or self-induced mental dysfunction would generate a health-care need. Certainly we can think of cases of mental dysfunctions that are attributable to dysfunctional families, and certainly we can think of combinations of biological dysfunctions and bad habits (Attention Deficit Disorder comes to mind here). In personal e-mail communication with Daniels (2/14/98), he indicates that personal responsibility is the key to disentangling this conundrum. Clearly, people are not responsible for either their genetic code or the families into which they are born. On the other hand, if they refuse to take responsibility for their disabilities (lingering neuroses, for example), then to insist on treatment would normally be unjustified paternalism.

19. Ibid, p. 28.

20. The World Health Organization takes health to be a 'state of complete physical, mental, and social well-being, and not merely the absence of

disease or infirmity.' From the Preamble to the Constitution of the World Health Organization. See Daniels, p. 29.

21. Green, p. 121.

22. Daniels, p. 29.

23. Ibid., 34.

24. Ibid., p. 31.

25. The range of opportunity also seems to be heavily influenced by social assumptions, e.g., that one may need breasts in order not to be seen as some sort of aberration in our sexist society. But, again, that seems to be a social need and not a need relative to biological functioning.

26. Daniels, p. 31.

27. In his discussion of the mastectomy patient, he appeals to Blue Cross/Blue Shield's decision to reverse their policy on mastectomies following a general outcry from the public upon refusal of restorative surgery.

28. Charlene Hoffman, National Center for Education Studies, e-mail address: http://nces.ed.gov/pubs/97384.html

29. The Twentieth Century Fund, *Medicare Reform: A Twentieth Century Fund Guide to the Issues* (New York: Twentieth Century Fund Press, 1995).

30. Daniels, N., (New York, NY: Cambridge University Press, 1996).

31. Ibid., p. 346.

32. Ibid., p. 346.

33. Ibid., p. 347.

Chapter 4

1. Walzer, Michael, *Spheres of Justice* (U. S., Basic Books, Inc., 1983).

2. The liberal individualist method of deciding upon principles in abstraction from actual communities is represented most clearly by Rawls, Daniels and Green.

3. See Mulhall and Swift in *Liberals and Communitarians* (Cambridge: Blackwell Publishers, 1992), p. 10 for a discussion on this.

4. Ibid., p. 8.

5. Ibid., p. 87.

6. Ibid.., p. 9.

7. Ibid., p. xiii.

8. Ibid., p. 83.

9. Ibid. , p. 8.

10. Ibid., p. 88.

11. Ibid., p. 75.

12. Ibid., p. 88.

13. Ibid., p. 88.

14. Ibid., p. 59.

15. Ibid., p. 90.

16. Ibid., p. 89.

17. Ronald Dworkin makes this same point in "To Each His Own," *New York Review of Books*, April 14, 1983, pp. 46-47.

18. Ibid., p. 65.

19. Ibid., p. 103.

20. Ibid. , p. 104.

21. Ibid., p. 47.

22. Georgia Warnke makes a point similar to this in *Justice and Interpretation* (Cambridge, MA: The MIT Press, 1993), pp. 18-19. Here, she is concerned that different groups of people in the US interpret the meaning of health care differently.

23. Ibid.

24. See Daniels, p. 106 in *Justice and Justification* for a discussion of this.

25. Walzer, p. 82.

26. Ibid. , p. 29.

27. I want to be clear that I do not mean "life plans" as Daniels means it. I do not include life plans outside of jobs and careers. On the other hand, I do believe that Daniels is correct in that we can't expect publicly provided health care to return individuals to plans of life they have already chosen (i.e., effective life plans), whether they be in the broad sense as Daniels means them, or in the narrow sense, as I mean them. If a democratically chosen package of health care fortuitously does return someone to her effective life plan, however, so much the better.

28. Joshua Cohen, review of *Spheres of Justice,* in *Journal of Philosophy* 83:3 (August 1986), 457-68.

Chapter 5

1. San Bernardino Sun, January 24, 1998, A4.

2. For instance, community colleges offer free of charge, flu vaccinations to their part-time faculty members who are not covered under an insurance scheme. Public schools do this as well, for their substitute teachers.

3. I am not denying here that medical care may be required for withdrawal from an addiction. Rather, I am suggesting that medical care is probably no more efficacious in the recovery process than 12-step programs. Most in-hospital treatment programs insist on participation in a 12-step

program for their patients to be considered in compliance with a treatment program.

4. This is a point made by Rawls in *Political Liberalism.* He insists, I think quite rightly, that the basic political structure must remain silent with respect to any particular moral, religious or comprehensive doctrine, since otherwise people will be forced to support doctrines to which they have strong disagreements. In turn, this circumstance will make for an unstable society.

5. Of course, there are many overlaps between publicly funded treatments and employment-based insurance. All that seems to indicate to me is that all humans have biological similarities, and that it is extremely difficult to draw hard and fast lines between the boundaries of different distributions.

6. I rejected the notion of "reasonable" preferences or life plans in the Daniels' chapter. But that was in connection with a state obligation. I think at the level of employment-based insurance, there is nothing wrong with reasonable preferences, since it simply gives an employer more leeway in health care insurance benefits.

7. Walzer, of course, rejects the free market principle as the proper criterion of distribution. Green and Daniels might make room for it on a second tier of health care provision provided this second tier does not increase costs at the basic level of distribution.

8. Ibid., p. 6, italics added. If we take "reasons" to mean principles, this passage seems to indicate that first comes the meanings of goods, and those meanings generate the appropriate principle.

9. Ibid., p. 10.

10. Ibid., p. 82.

11. Ibid., p. 6.

Chapter 6

1. There is a good amount of discussion now whether people over the age of sixty-five and who have a good income, should qualify for Medicare

benefits. Another way we might deal with people on Medicare is to qualify them for health care under the principle of merit, since they have in the past contributed to the economic well-being of the nation. We might also think of the dependents of employees in this regard too. In some sense, the family unit supports the worker. It is conventional wisdom that a man without a wife and family will not rise above middle-management in his career. Presumably, either this circumstance will hold in the future for women as well, or men's success won't be dependent on marriage and a family.

2. Presumably, under conditions of great economic prosperity even treatments such as breast enhancement might be publicly covered if they improve an individual's chances for some life plan.

3. This assumes that in line with public provision, those who refuse to accept some responsibility for their treatment are eventually refused treatment.

4. The line between controversial treatments and quackery is not easy to draw. New procedures have been thought to be quackery, and instead turned out to be highly effective. On the other hand, procedures thought to be quackery, have turned out to be just that. And I am not convinced that peer review is always the best measure of drawing a line since "tried and true" procedures become entrenched in any field, making professionals overly cautious, sometimes, about accepting new treatments.

5. This is not to say that infertility does not affect other social goals. Certainly, the goal of having a family is affected. But in line with a Rawlsian conception of justice, I believe that while it may be unfortunate that an individual cannot conceive, it is nonetheless not a concern of the state if one cannot.

6. It is extremely difficult to characterize the sense in which I, or anyone else for that matter, mean "natural." I suppose I mean "natural" in a very intuitive sense that given our biology, it is not surprising that a certain condition may arise. For instance, given our physical make up it is not surprising that people get the flu after exposure to a virus. However, it would be surprising, indeed, if a plant got the flu after exposure to a virus, given its physical make up.

7. The slipperiness of the term "natural" can be seen in the following examples: events that occur in nature such as leaves falling off deciduous trees in the autumn follow the laws of cause and effect found in nature: there is a regularity to these events such that we can count on them to happen. It might be thought by "natural" that some people prefer living in a desert, but in order to do so, they must use unnatural methods such as air conditioning and diverting water from sources quite far away. It might be thought by some people that arising at 6:00 a.m. is natural, while other people naturally want to stay up most of the night, and arise after 10:00 a.m. It might be considered natural that grass grows, but hybrids of grass and cutting it down would be unnatural. It might be thought that motherhood comes naturally to a woman, but many young women take classes in parenting. These few examples suggest that the notion of "natural" is very elastic, and most of us do not know what we mean when we use the term, or at least we use it in so many ways that it does not possess a firm meaning.

8. The San Bernardino Sun, Feb. 8, 1998, A3. A bill was sent to Governor Wilson which would require that health plans include contraceptives just as they cover other prescriptive drugs (about two-thirds of them exclude contraceptives). The basis of this argument is that because of this exclusion, women pay 68 percent more than men in out-of-pocket expenses for health care (according to the Women's Research and Education Institute in Washington).

9. Jane English makes this point in "Abortion and the Concept of the Person," in *Moral Controversies*, pp. 3-32.

10. *Dority v. Superior Court of San Bernardino County*, 193 Cal. Rptr. 287 (Cal. App. 4 Dist. 1983).

11. These tests were in accord with the proper medical procedures for determining brain death.

12. Loma Linda defines brain death as total and irreversible cessation of brain function, including the brain stem.

13. *Dority v. Superior Court of San Bernardino County.*

14. Ibid.

15. Health and Safety Code section 7185.

16. Ibid.

17. Ibid., where the competent patient's right to instruct the physician to withhold or withdraw treatment is based on a fundamental right to privacy, the courts must show a compelling state interest in order to override such a right.

18. Steven H. Miles, "Informed Demand for 'Non-Beneficial Medical Treatment," in *Ethical Issues in Modern Medicine*, eds. John Arras and Bonnie Steinbock (Mountain View, CA: Mayfield Publishing Co., 1995), pp. 277-280.

19. Tom Beauchamp and James Childress, *Principles of Biomedical Ethics* (New York: Oxford University Press, 1994), p. 519.

20. Bonnie Steinbock, "The Lakeberg Siamese Twins: When is Treatment Futile?," in *Ethical Issues in Modern Medicine*, (Mountain View, CA: Mayfield Publishing Company, 1995), pp. 276-277.

21. Charles Fried, *Right and Wrong* (Cambridge, MA: Harvard University Press, 1978), Chapter 5.

22. The Press-Enterprise. May 12, 1996, section B.

23. Mary McGrory, The Press-Enterprise, "Americans are Faced With a Tough Decision: What Kind of People Will They Become?" A-5, 1994.

BIBLIOGRAPHY

Banfield, Eric, *A Heartland Perspective: The Folly of Employer-Based Health Insurance,* The Heartland Institute (Westmont, IL), August 17, 1994.

Beauchamp, Tom and James Childress, *Principles of Biomedical Ethics* (New York: Oxford University press, 1994).

Blendon, R. J., K. Donelan, C. A. Hill, W. Carter, D. Beatrice, D. Altman, "Paying Medical Bills in the United States: Why Health Insurance Isn't Enough," *The Journal of the American Medical Association*, 1994.

Braybrooke, David, "Let Needs Diminish that Preferences May Prosper," *Studies in Moral Philosophy* in *American Philosophical Quarterly Monograph*, Series, No. 1, (Oxford: Blackwells, 1968).

Cal. Rptr. 287 (Cal. App. 4 Dist. 1983).

California Safety Code, section 7185.

Cohen, Joshua, "Review of *Spheres of Justice*," in *Journal of Philosophy* 83:3 (August 1986).

Daniels, Norman, *Just Health Care* (Cambridge, Mass.: Cambridge University Press, 1985).

———, *Justice and Justification* (Cambridge, Mass.: Cambridge University Press, 1996).

Dworkin, Ronald, "To Each His Own," *New York Review of Books*, April 14, 1983.

English, Jane, "Abortion and the Concept of the Person," in Steven Jay Gold, ed., *Moral Controversies* (Wadsworth Publishing, 1993).

Fried, Charles, *Right and Wrong* (Cambridge, MA.: Harvard University Press, 1978).

Green, Ronald, "Health Care and Justice in Contract Theory Perspective," in Robert Veatch and Roy Branson (eds), *Ethics and Health Policy* (Cambridge, Mass.: Ballinger, 1976).

Health Care Financing Administration: Data from the Office of National Health Statistics. Office of Personal Management.

Health Resources and Services Administration. *The Hill-Burton Uncompensated Services Program: A Profile.* Rockville, MD: Health Resources and Services Administration, 1994.

Kymlicka Will, *Contemporary Political Philosophy* (New York: Oxford University Press, 1990).

McCloskey, J. H., "Human Needs, Rights, and Political Values," *American Philosophical Quarterly,* 13:1.

Michelman, Frank, "Constitutional Welfare Rights and *A Theory of Justice*, " in N. Daniels (ed.) *Reading Rawls*, (Stanford University Press, 1989).

Miles, Steven H., "Informed Demand for 'Non-Beneficial Medical Treatment," in John Arras and Bonnie Steinbock (eds.) *Ethical Issues in Modern Medicine*, (Mountain View, CA: Mayfield Publishing Co., 1995).

Mulhall, Stephen and Adam Swift, *Liberals & Communitarians* (Cambridge: Blackwell Publishers, 1992).

Press-Enterprise (1996).

———(1994).

Rawls, John, *A Theory of Justice* (Cambridge, Mass.: The Belknap Press of Harvard University Press, 1971).

———, *Political Liberalism* (New York: Columbia University Press, 1993).

———, "Social Unity and Primary Goods," in A. Sen and B. Williams (eds.) *Utilitarianism and Beyond* (Cambridge, MA: Cambridge University Press, 1982).

San Bernardino Sun (January 1998).

———, (February 1998).

Steinbock, Bonnie, "The Lakeberg Siamese Twins: When is Treatment Futile?" in *Ethical Issues in Modern Medicine*, eds. John Arras and Bonnie Steinbock (Mountain View, CA: Mayfield Publishing Company, 1995).

Twentieth Century Fund, *Medicare Reform: A Twentieth Century Fund Guide to the Issues* (New York: Twentieth Century Fund Press, 1995).

Urban Institute (1995).

Walzer, Michael, *Spheres of Justice* (U.S.: Basic Books, 1983).

Warnke, Georgia, *Justice and Interpretation* (Cambridge, MA: The MIT Press, 1993).

Weissman, Joel, "Uncompensated Hospital Care," in *The Journal of the American Medical Association,* September 11, 1996, vol. 276, No. 10.

———, Lukas Van Deusen, A. M. Epstein, "Bad Debt and Free Care in Massachusetts Hospitals: The Role of the Uninsured and Underinsured Patients," in *Health Affairs*, Summer 1992; 11.

Williams, Bernard, "The Idea of Equality," in H.A. Bedau (ed.), *Justice and Equality*, (Englewood Cliffs, NJ: Prentice-Hall), 1971.

World Health Organization, *Official Record of World Health Organization* 2, No. 100, July 1946.

INTERNATIONAL HEALTHCARE ETHICS

Issues in healthcare ethics affect almost every person all over the world. The immense leaps in science and technology, changes in the general perception of national and global interests, possible limits in resources, mass communication, and other factors have currently engendered a stronger interest and concern with health. This may range from the commonly discussed issues of euthanasia, abortion, macro- and microallocation of resources, and mandatory AIDS testing to the less frequently addressed but still vital issues in pharmacology, genetic testing, screening and therapy, nursing, mental health, and public health.

Books, articles, and scholarly studies appear frequently in many countries. In each, the literature tends to consider the ethics of healthcare issues in depth but from a standpoint defined by culture and nationality, and by national government policies and perspectives. Such a standpoint necessarily limits and excludes many potentially useful and innovative approaches to issues. The International Healthcare Ethics Series presents a broad perspective on a wide range of healthcare issues to stimulate thought and the exchange of ideas between cultures and nations. It also offers a forum for addressing healthcare issues that can affect each of us on a global scale. Manuscripts are welcome from universities, bioethics centers, and healthcare organizations.

For additional information about this series or for the submission of manuscripts, please contact:

Peter Lang Publishing, Inc.
Acquisitions Department
516 N. Charles St., 2nd Floor
Baltimore, MD 21201

To order other books in this series, please contact our Customer Service Department:

(800) 770-LANG (within the U.S.)
(212) 647-7706 (outside the U.S.)
(212) 647-7707 FAX

or browse online by series:

WWW.PETERLANGUSA.COM